Study Guide to Accompa

CLINICAL DRUG THERAPY

RATIONALES FOR NURSING PRACTICE

Fifth Edition

Gail Ropelewski-Ryan, RN, MSN (Professor)
Nurse Education, Health, Physical Education and Recreation
Corning Community College
Corning, New York

Anne Collins Abrams, RN, MSN (Associate Professor)
Department of Baccalaureate and Graduate Nursing
College of Allied Health and Nursing
Eastern Kentucky University
Richmond, Kentucky

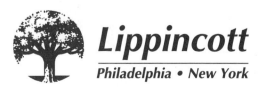

Lippincott

Philadelphia • New York

Acquisition Editor: Margaret Zuccarini
Assistant Editor: Sara Lauber
Ancillary Editor: Doris S. Wray
Production Manager: Helen Ewan
Production Editor: Virginia Barishek
Production Service: Berliner Inc.
Printer/Binder: Victor Graphics

Fifth edition

ISBN: 0-397-55373-0

Care has been taken to confirm the accuracy of the information presented and to describe generally accepted practices. However, the authors, editors, and publisher are not responsible for errors or omissions or for any consequences from application of the information in this book and make no warranty, express or implied, with respect to the contents of the publication.

The authors, editors and publisher have exerted every effort to ensure that drug selection and dosage set forth in this text are in accordance with current recommendations and practice at the time of publication. However, in view of ongoing research, changes in government regulations, and the constant flow of information relating to drug therapy and drug reactions, the reader is urged to check the package insert for each drug for any change in indications and dosages and for added warnings and precautions. This is particularly important when the recommended agent is a new or infrequently employed drug.

INTRODUCTION

The *Study Guide to Accompany Clinical Drug Therapy: Rationales for Nursing Practice,* fifth edition, has been developed to complement Anne Abrams' text. It provides a wealth of learning opportunities to reinforce content that students have read in the text and to promote their ability to apply this information in the patient care setting.

Pharmacology is a tough and demanding science, fraught with seemingly limitless detail about an ever-growing number of drugs. Helping students learn the principles of pharmacology as applied to nursing practice to foster safe and effective management of drug therapy is perhaps one of the most challenging tasks surrounding nursing education today.

The *Study Guide* offers a variety of activities that incorporate approaches to learning designed to accommodate many student learning styles and increase the appeal of learning. The exercises have been chosen to help students establish a connection between how a drug works and why it is used for a particular disorder.

The *Study Guide* will help prepare students in the following ways:

- *Prepare for NCLEX test-taking:*
  NCLEX-style multiple-choice questions in every chapter give students an opportunity to practice their test-taking skills.

- *Develop critical thinking skills:*
  Case study exercises challenge students to develop their critical thinking skills and help students explore how they would apply those skills in a clinical situation.

- *Develop insight about client teaching needs:*
  Each exercise is aimed at expanding the students' knowledge base and understanding of drug therapy and increasing students' understanding of what patients need to know to maximize their drug therapy. Students will use information from the text to develop a teaching plan for persons who will require medication when they return home.

- *Receive immediate reinforcement of learning:*
  Answers for the multiple-choice questions and exercises are provided in the back of the workbook, allowing immediate feedback about the correctness of exercise answers.

- *Expand personal understanding of drug therapy:*
  Completing the exercises and working through the case studies provides valuable opportunity for students to immediately enhance learning effectiveness, building on classroom lectures, textbook reading and reflection, and completion of exercises provided at the end of each text chapter.

Contents

INTRODUCTION TO DRUG THERAPY

1

Introduction to Pharmacology

MATCHING EXERCISE

Terms and Concepts

Match the concept with the term for it.

1. _____ The study of drugs.

2. _____ An individual drug that represents a group of drugs.

3. _____ Chemicals that change functions of living organisms.

4. _____ A group of drugs with common characteristics or uses.

5. _____ The law which regulates distribution of narcotics and other drugs of abuse.

6. _____ Studies to determine potential uses and adverse effects.

7. _____ A chemical mediator.

8. _____ Related to the chemical name; often indicates the drug group.

9. _____ Designated by the manufacturer.

10. _____ There is an increased number during allergic reactions.

11. _____ The first federal law which established standards for drug products.

12. _____ An important mechanism for transporting protein into cells.

13. _____ A mechanism for secreting intracellular substances into extracellular spaces.

14. _____ An adverse effect involving the liver.

15. _____ Results in edema and impaired cellular function.

A. Drugs.

B. Controlled Substances Act.

C. Eosinophils.

D. Pharmacology.

E. Prototype.

F. Generic name.

G. Drug classification.

H. Trade name.

I. Histamine.

J. Pure Food and Drug Act.

K. Clinical trials.

L. Exocytosis.

M. Hepatotoxicity.

N. Cellular injury.

O. Pinocytosis.

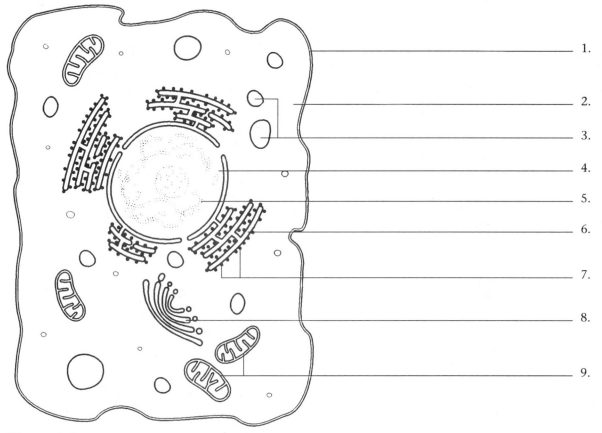

Figure 1-1

FILL IN THE BLANK

Cell Physiology, Part I

Fill in the blanks in Figure 1-1 with the terms below.

Golgi apparatus   Cell membrane

Cytoplasm   Mitochondria

Endoplasmic reticulum   Chromatin

Nucleus   Lysosomes

Ribosomes

Cell Physiology, Part II

1. Explain the relationship between the physiology of a body cell and the pharmacodynamics of a drug.

REVIEW QUESTIONS

1. The chemical name given to a drug that is independent of the manufacturer who holds the patent.
   a. Generic name.
   b. Brand name.
   c. Trade name.
   d. Family name.

2. Most drugs today are derived from
   a. plants.
   b. animals.
   c. synthetic compounds.
   d. minerals.

3. A molecule that, when manipulated, produces a genetically identical molecule is referred to as a
   a. clone.
   b. gene.
   c. hybrid.
   d. encoded protein.

4. Hormones and other substances are produced by the
   a. mitochondria.
   b. cytoplasm.
   c. endoplasmic reticulum.
   d. Golgi complex.

5. During which phase of drug trials are drugs administered to healthy volunteers?
   a. Phase IV.
   b. Phase III.
   c. Phase II.
   d. Phase I.

6. The standard by which other drugs within a classification are compared.
   a. Prototype.
   b. Provisional model.
   c. Proximal model.
   d. Prototroph.

7. The following medication has been transferred from prescription to nonprescription status:
   a. Cimetidine (Tagamet).
   b. Acetaminophen (Tylenol).
   c. Codeine.
   d. Diazepam (Valium).

8. The body's main defense against pathogenic bacteria is a group of leukocytes called
   a. nongranulocytes.
   b. basophils.
   c. eosinophils.
   d. neutrophils.

9. Nutrients are broken down by
   a. bradykinin.
   b. enzymes.
   c. exocytosis.
   d. kinins.

10. The first law to require proof of safety before a new drug could be marketed was the
    a. Pure Food and Drug Act of 1906.
    b. Kefauver–Harris Amendment of 1962.
    c. Food, Drug and Cosmetic Act of 1938.
    d. Drug Regulation and Reform Act of 1978.

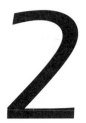 **2**

Basic Concepts and Processes

FILL IN THE BLANKS

Complete the following sentences.

1. Drug movement and drug action are affected by a drug's ability to _____.

2. _____ soluble drugs cross cell membranes more easily than _____ soluble drugs.

3. _____ is a major determinant of a drug's bioavailability.

4. For most drugs, the presence of food in the stomach _____ the rate of absorption.

5. Besides the stomach, other absorptive sites include _____ and _____.

6. Distribution depends largely on the _____.

7. An important factor in drug distribution is _____.

8. Only the free or _____ portion of a drug acts on body cells.

9. The _____ regulates diffusion of drug molecules from the bloodstream into brain tissue.

10. _____ is the method by which drugs are inactivated or biotransformed by the body.

11. Most drugs are metabolized by _____ in the _____.

12. Some drugs stimulate liver cells to produce larger amounts of drug metabolizing enzymes. This is referred to as _____.

13. Organs of excretion include the _____, _____, _____, and _____.

14. Receptors that bind with drugs include _____, _____, and nucleic acids.

15. Only drugs able to chemically _____ to the receptors in a particular body tissue can exert _____ effects on that tissue.

16. The _____ available to interact with drug molecules also affects the extent of drug action.

17. A drug's _____ affects its ability to reach tissue fluids.

18. Route of _____ affects drug actions and responses by influencing _____ and _____.

19. Drug actions may be more pronounced in _____, _____, and older adults because of their _____ and _____ function.

20. Rapid development of tolerance after only a few doses is called _____.

DEFINITIONS

Define each of the following terms.

1. Passive diffusion.

   _____

2. Active transport.

   _____

3. Excretion.

   _____

4. Serum half-life.

   _____

5. Agonists.

   _____

6. Antagonists.

   _____

7. Synergism.

   _____

8. Idiosyncracy.

   _____

MATCHING EXERCISE

Terms and Concepts

Match the concept with the term for it.

1. _____ Food ingested with oral medications.
2. _____ Coumadin.
3. _____ MAO inhibitor.
4. _____ Tetracycline.

A. Combines with calcium in milk to form an insoluble compound.

B. Slows absorption and gastric emptying.

C. Food high in vitamin K will decrease its effect.

D. Ingestion of food high in tyramine and this drug can cause hypertension.

REVIEW QUESTIONS

1. Your client tells you that 5 years ago she had penicillin and developed hives. Based on this information you will

   a. administer the penicillin as ordered and observe for a reaction.

   b. administer the penicillin with an antihistamine to avert a reaction.

   c. withhold the penicillin and contact her physician.

   d. administer the penicillin intramuscularly to avoid gastric absorption.

2. Taking erythromycin with food will

   a. enhance the rate of absorption.

   b. prolong the therapeutic effect.

   c. decrease the rate of elimination.

   d. delay the rate of absorption.

3. Following a diagnosis of meningitis, the physician ordered penicillin G for your client. This drug was selected because it is

   a. fat soluble and able to cross the blood–brain barrier.

   b. water soluble and crosses the blood–brain barrier in the presence of inflammation.

   c. transported to the brain via active transport.

   d. one of the few drugs that uses passive diffusion to reach the brain.

4. You admit a chronic alcoholic with Crohn's disease and peripheral edema who smokes two packages of cigarettes a day. You will assess him for possible toxic drug effects primarily related to

   a. decreased lung capacity.

   b. impaired liver function.

   c. decreased cardiac output.

   d. impaired absorption.

5. Your client, who has been using nitroglycerin for 5 years, complains that it does not work as it used to. This is an example of

   a. supersensitivity.

   b. an agonist response.

   c. tolerance.

   d. an idiosyncracy.

6. Your client's lab work indicates hypoalbuminemia. This can result in

   a. decreased drug metabolism.

   b. prolonged half-life of a medication.

   c. excess free drug and an exaggerated effect.

   d. a reduced therapeutic effect.

7. Your client is to be started on warfarin (Coumadin). She has been taking aspirin daily for arthritis for 5 years. You notify her physician of this because

   a. aspirin increases platelet aggregation.

   b. aspirin displaces Coumadin from the binding site, increasing bleeding potential.

   c. aspirin creates an acidic environment, which inhibits Coumadin absorption.

   d. Coumadin administered with aspirin results in excessive clotting.

8. Which of the following statements is true regarding the half-life of medications?

   a. Increasing the dose will increase the half-life of the medication.

   b. Five half-lives are usually required for a medication to be completely excreted.

   c. Clients with renal disease usually have decreased drug half-lives.

   d. The half-life of a drug determines how often the drug is to be administered.

9. All of the following will affect a client's response to medications *except*

   a. psychological state.

   b. climate.

   c. body weight.

   d. age.

10. Your client, who is being treated with a MAO inhibitor for depression, ate aged cheese and wine for dinner. She will likely have the following response:

    a. Severe headache.

    b. Diarrhea.

    c. Decreased urinary output.

    d. No ill effects.

3

Administering Medications

MATCHING EXERCISES

Terms and Concepts

Match the concept with the term for it.

1. _____ An acceptable site for IM injections.

2. _____ Both eyes.

3. _____ Narcotic analgesics and other drugs with potential for abuse.

4. _____ One ounce.

5. _____ Before meals.

6. _____ Units of measurements in the metric system.

7. _____ IV, IM, SC injections.

8. _____ Glass containers that may contain one or several doses.

9. _____ An acceptable site for SC injections.

10. _____ Under the tongue.

11. _____ Glass containers that contain approximately one dose of a drug.

12. _____ The vastus lateralis muscle is a commonly used location for IM injection in this group.

13. _____ An anatomical landmark for administering an injection in the deltoid muscle.

14. _____ A drug preparation suitable for use in the eye.

15. _____ A dosage form designed to dissolve in the small intestine rather than in the stomach.

16. _____ A drug preparation suitable for use in the ear.

17. _____ Applied to the skin.

18. _____ Administration of this medication requires the use of a special syringe.

19. _____ Physicians administer medication in this location.

20. _____ A suppository can be administered here.

A. Controlled drugs.

B. Ventrogluteal.

C. 30 ml.

D. a.c.

E. Meter, gram, liter.

F. OU.

G. Parenteral.

H. Vials.

I. Abdomen.

J. Sublingual.

K. Topical.

L. Ampules.

M. Acromion process.

N. Ophthalmic solution.

O. Children.

P. Enteric coated.

Q. 240 ml.

R. Otic.

S. Insulin.

T. Demerol.

U. Intrathecal.

V. Intravaginally.

Abbreviations

Match each abbreviation (numbered items) with its definition (lettered items). Each definition may be used only once.

1. _____ q.d.
2. _____ PRN.
3. _____ q.i.d.
4. _____ stat.
5. _____ qlh.
6. _____ h.s.
7. _____ IM.
8. _____ SL.
9. _____ PO.
10. _____ OD.

A. Right eye.
B. Intramuscular.
C. Immediately.
D. Sublingual.
E. Bedtime.
F. When needed.
G. Four times daily.
H. Oral.
I. Once daily.
J. Every hour.

Equivalents

Match each quantity (numbered items) with its equivalent (lettered items). Each equivalent may be used only once.

1. _____ 0.6 g.
2. _____ 60, 64, or 65 mg.
3. _____ 1000 ml.
4. _____ 8 oz.
5. _____ 300 mg.
6. _____ 650 mg.
7. _____ 30 ml.
8. _____ 5 ml.
9. _____ 2.2 lb.
10. _____ 1 liter.

A. 0.3 g.
B. 30 cc.
C. 1 gr.
D. 10 gr.
E. 600 mg.
F. 1 tsp.
G. 1 kg.
H. 1 liter.
I. 1 lb.
J. 1 tbsp.
K. 250 ml.
L. 1 quart.

DIAGRAM

Subcutaneous Injections

Mark on Figure 3-1 where subcutaneous injections can be administered.

PRACTICE QUESTIONS

Medication Orders

1. The physician's order reads: Administer ASA p.c. What time will you give the medication?
   a. 10 P.M.
   b. 9 A.M.
   c. 8 A.M., 1 P.M., 6 P.M.
   d. 7 A.M., 11 A.M., 4 P.M.

2. The physician's order reads: Administer Maalox at a.c. and h.s. When will you administer the medication?
   a. 7 A.M., 11 A.M., 4 P.M., 9 P.M.
   b. 9 A.M., 9 P.M.
   c. 10 A.M., 2 P.M., 6 P.M., 10 P.M.
   d. 7 A.M., 7 P.M.

3. The physician's order reads: Administer furosemide (Lasix) b.i.d. You will administer it
   a. daily.
   b. every other day.
   c. twice a day.
   d. on odd days.

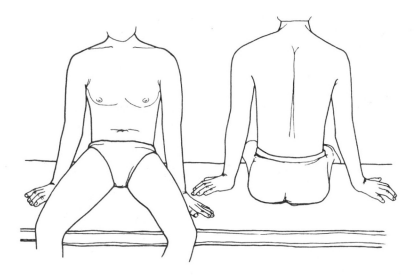

Figure 3-1

DOSAGE CALCULATIONS

Practice Set I

1. Order: Ferrous sulfate 600 mg PO.
   Label: Ferrous sulfate 325 mg/tablet.
   Administer:

   _____

2. Order: Penicillin 250,000 units IV.
   Label: Penicillin 20 million units in 20 ml.
   Administer:

   _____

3. Order: KCl 40 mEq PO.
   Label: KCl 10 mEq/15 ml.
   Administer:

   _____

4. Order: Digoxin 0.375 mg PO.
   Label: Digoxin 0.125 mg/tablet.
   Administer:

   _____

5. Order: Atropine 0.2 mg IM.
   Label: Atropine 0.4 mg/cc.
   Administer:

   _____

6. Order: Demerol 30 mg IM.
   Label: Demerol 75 mg/cc.
   Administer:

   _____

7. Order: Gentamicin 50 mg IV.
   Label: Gentamicin 80 mg/2 ml.
   Administer:

   _____

8. Order: Aminophylline 0.4 g IV.
   Label: Aminophylline 500 mg/10 cc.
   Administer:

   _____

9. Order: Heparin 4000 units IV.
   Label: Heparin 1000 unit/ml.
   Administer:

   _____

10. Order: Digoxin 0.125 mg IM.
    Label: Digoxin 0.5 mg/2 cc.
    Administer:

    _____

Practice Set II

1. Two ounces are equivalent to how many milliliters?

   _____

2. The physician writes an order for 1 gram of
   aspirin. Each tablet contains 5 grains. How many
   tablets will you administer?

   _____

3. Mr. J. is to receive 12 ounces of magnesium citrate. How many milliliters should he receive?

   _____

4. Mr. P. weighs 132 lb. How many kilograms does
   he weigh?

   _____

5. You want Mrs. S. to drink 1.25 liters of solution.
   How many milliliters is she expected to drink?

   _____

6. The physician writes an order for 125 mg. The bottle is marked 50 mg/ml. How many milliliters will you administer?

   _____

7. The order reads administer 20 grains. On hand you have grams. How many grams will you administer?

   _____

8. An ampule contains 50 mg of a drug in 2 ml of solution. The physician orders 10 mg of the drug. How many milliliters will you administer?

   _____

9. The order reads administer 2500 units of heparin SC. The vial contains 10,000 units/ml. How many milliliters will you administer?

   _____

10. The order reads give 10 ml of a solution. Mrs. J. wants to know how many teaspoons or tablespoons this equals. The best answer would be:

    _____

REVIEW QUESTIONS

Dosage Calculations

1. Order: Aspirin 5 gr PO.
   Label: Aspirin 325 mg/tablet.
   Administer:
   a. 1 tablet.
   b. 1½ tablet.
   c. 2 tablets.
   d. 2½ tablets.

2. Order: Penicillin 500,000 units IV.
   Label: Penicillin 20 million units in 20 ml.
   Administer:
   a. 0.5 ml.
   b. 1 ml.
   c. 1.5 ml.
   d. 2 ml.

3. Order: KCl 20 mEq PO.
   Label: KCl 10 mEq/15 ml.
   Administer:
   a. 10 ml.
   b. 15 ml.
   c. 20 ml.
   d. 30 ml.

4. Order: Digoxin 0.25 mg PO.
   Label: Digoxin 0.125 mg/tablet.
   Administer:
   a. 1 tablet.
   b. 2 tablets.
   c. 4 tablets.
   d. 5 tablets.

5. Order: Atropine 0.6 mg IM.
   Label: Atropine 0.4 mg/cc.
   Administer:
   a. 0.75 cc.
   b. 1.25 cc.
   c. 1.50 cc.
   d. 1.75 cc.

6. Order: Demerol 30 mg IM.
   Label: Demerol 100 mg/cc.
   Administer:
   a. 0.3 cc.
   b. 0.4 cc.
   c. 0.5 cc.
   d. 0.6 cc.

7. Order: Heparin 2500 units SC.
   Label: Heparin 10,000 units/ml.
   Administer:
   a. 0.25 ml.
   b. 0.5 ml.
   c. 0.75 ml.
   d. 1 ml.

8. Order: Gentamicin 65 mg IV.
   Label: Gentamicin 80 mg/2 ml.
   Administer:
   a. 1.5 ml.
   b. 1.6 ml.
   c. 1.3 ml.
   d. 1.4 ml.

9. Order: Aminophylline 0.5 g IV.
   Label: Aminophylline 500 mg/10 cc.
   Administer:
   a. 1 cc.
   b. 10 cc.
   c. 100 cc.
   d. 1000 cc.

10. Order: Heparin 2000 units IV.
    Label: Heparin 1000 unit/ml.
    Administer:
    a. 1 ml.
    b. 2 ml.
    c. 3 ml.
    d. 4 ml.

4

Nursing Process in Drug Therapy

TRUE OR FALSE

1. _____ When effective, it is generally better to use as few drugs in as low doses as possible.

2. _____ Fixed-dose combinations of two or three drugs are preferred over two or three single drugs, when available.

3. _____ Clients with severe renal disease often need smaller-than-average doses of drugs that are excreted by the kidney.

4. _____ Some drugs can be given safely during pregnancy.

5. _____ The preferred site for IM injection in infants is the thigh.

6. _____ The most accurate method of calculating drug dosages for children is a method based on age.

7. _____ Drug therapy in newborn infants must be very cautious because of immature liver and kidney functions.

8. _____ Adverse drug effects are more likely to occur in elderly clients than in young or middle-aged adults.

9. _____ Newer drugs are more effective than older ones.

10. _____ The nurse should assess the client's condition before giving PRN medications.

11. _____ Drugs with long half-lives may not reach maximum therapeutic effect for several days or weeks.

12. _____ Older adults have decreased amounts of body fat so fat-soluble drugs have a shorter duration of action.

13. _____ Decreased serum protein levels can result in increased serum concentration and increased risk of adverse effects.

14. _____ When doing a medication history the nurse should also ask about nonprescription drug use including alcohol, caffeine, and nicotine.

15. _____ A client's renal function should be considered before drug therapy is started.

CRITICAL THINKING CASE STUDY

Pediatric Calculations

M., a 5-year-old, is admitted to your unit with a seizure disorder. M. weighs 44 lb. The recommended dosage range of phenobarbital is 4–6 mg/kg/day for anticonvulsant effects.

1. Identify the maximum daily dosage.

   _____

2. If the above amount is to be given in three equal doses, what is the amount (mg) per dose?

   _____

3. The pharmacy sends you a phenobarbital solution containing 15 mg/ml. How many milliliters are needed for each dose calculated above?

   _____

M. is to be started on phenytoin (Dilantin) The recommended dosage range of phenytoin (Dilantin) is 4–7 mg/kg/day. The pharmacy sends a solution of 100 mg/2 ml.

4. Identify the minimum daily dose (mg).

   _____

5. Identify the maximum daily dose (mg).

   _____

6. You are to administer the maximum daily dose to M. in two equal doses. Identify the amount needed (ml) for each dose.

   _____

M. is complaining of pain. The physician orders 6 mg of morphine subcutaneously q6h. The recommended dosage range of morphine for a child is 0.1–0.2 mg/kg.

7. Identify where you would administer the medication.

_____

8. Determine whether the dose ordered for M. is acceptable, and discuss what you do.

_____

OBTAINING A MEDICATION HISTORY

Using the following form, select a patient, friend, or family member and obtain his or her medication history.

Name _____ Age _____

Occupation _____ Educational level _____

Health problems, acute and chronic

Do you have any allergies?

If yes, describe specific effects or symptoms.

Part I. Prescription medications

Do you take any prescription medications on a regular basis?

If yes, ask the following about each medication:

Name: _____ Dose: _____

Frequency: _____ Specific times: _____

How long taken: _____ Reason for use: _____
Are you able to take this medicine pretty much as prescribed?

What do you do when you miss a dose of medication?

Does anyone else help you take your medication?

What information or instructions were you given when the medication was first prescribed?

Do you think the medication is doing what it was prescribed to do?

Have you had any problems that you attribute to the medication?

Do you take any prescription medications on an irregular basis?

If yes, ask the following about each medication:

Name: _____   Reason: _____

Dose: _____   How long taken: _____

Frequency: _____

Part II. Nonprescription medications

Do you take any OTC medications for the following problems?

| | MEDICATION | | | |
PROBLEM	Yes/No	Name	Amount	Frequency
Pain				
Headache				
Sleep				
Cold				
Indigestion				
Heartburn				
Diarrhea				
Constipation				
Other				

Part III. Social habits

	Yes/No	Amount
Coffee (decaffeinated, regular)		
Tea (decaffeinated, regular)		
Soda (decaffeinated, regular, sugar-free)		
Alcohol		
Tobacco		
Candy (chocolates, licorice, diet candy)		

Part IV. Physicians

Name	What you see them for	Phone #
_____	_____	_____
_____	_____	_____
_____	_____	_____
_____	_____	_____

REVIEW QUESTIONS

1. A 90-year-old is started on digoxin (Lanoxin); because of the client's age, the dosage of this medication may need to be adjusted due to his:

   a. increased body fat.

   b. decreased gastrointestinal secretions.

   c. decreased glomerular filtration rate.

   d. lack of ability to metabolize drugs.

2. A 3-month-old is receiving a topical steroid; because of the increased absorption of topical drugs in infants, you should assess for

   a. increased elimination of other medications.

   b. fluid volume overload.

   c. decreased urinary output.

   d. suppressed adrenal cortical function.

3. The following physiologic characteristic of the elderly may increase the serum concentrations of drugs that are bound to protein:

   a. Decreased cardiac output.

   b. Decreased serum albumin.

   c. Decreased liver enzymes.

   d. Decreased number of functioning nephrons.

4. S., age 6, refuses to take her antibiotic. To proceed, you should

   a. hold S. down, open her mouth, and administer the medication.

   b. tell S. you will administer the medication by injection if she does not cooperate.

   c. mix the medication with a favorite food or fluid to make it more acceptable.

   d. call S.'s mother and ask her to come in and assist you.

5. Which of the following statements is true in regards to the administration of water-soluble drugs in infants as compared to adults?

   a. A smaller portion of the infant's body is water; therefore, the infant requires smaller dosages.

   b. A larger portion of the infants body is water; therefore, the infant requires larger doses of water soluble drugs.

   c. A smaller portion of the infants body is fat; therefore, the infant requires a larger dose of water soluble drugs.

   d. A larger portion of the infants body is water, but usually a smaller dose is needed.

6. A 75-year-old client has just received an initial dose of lithium. Because of his total body water composition you would expect that the onset of action of lithium will

   a. be rapid and result in higher plasma concentrations.

   b. take longer and the duration will be prolonged.

   c. be rapid and the duration of action will be cut in half.

   d. be prolonged and result in lower plasma concentrations.

7. Before administering medications to a 9-month-old, the nurse should be aware that his or her decreased capacity for biotransformation of drugs will

   a. reduce blood levels of certain drugs.

   b. slow the metabolism and elimination of certain drugs.

   c. significantly limit the types of medications that can be administered.

   d. decrease the possibility of drug toxicity.

8. When digoxin (Lanoxin) is initially started, a relatively large dose is administered. This is referred to as a

   a. therapeutic dose.

   b. loading dose.

   c. maintenance dose.

   d. fixed dose.

9. The percentage of body water of an infant is

   a. 20–30%.

   b. 30–40%.

   c. 50–60%.

   d. 70–80%.

10. A 4-year-old child, weighing 22.8 kg, is to receive ampicillin (Omnipen). The adult dose is 450 mg q6h. Using Clark's rule (weight in pounds ÷ 150) × Adult dose = Child dose, determine the appropriate dose.

    a. 100 mg.

    b. 150 mg.

    c. 200 mg.

    d. 250 mg.

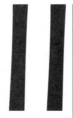

DRUGS
AFFECTING THE
CENTRAL
NERVOUS SYSTEM

5

Physiology of the Central Nervous System

FILL IN THE BLANK

Complete the following sentences.

1. The central nervous system is composed of the
   _____ and _____.

2. A _____ is a microscopic gap
   that separates _____.

3. Neurotransmitter substances include
   _____, _____
   (dopamine), (_____),
   _____, _____,
   _____, and _____.

4. The cerebral cortex is involved in all
   _____.

5. The thalamus receives impulses carrying sensa-
   tions such as _____,
   _____, _____,
   and _____.

6. The hypothalamus regulates _____,
   _____, _____,
   and _____.

7. The medulla oblongata contains neurons that
   form the vital _____,
   _____, and _____
   centers.

8. When stimulated, the reticular formation produces _____ and
   _____.

9. The limbic system regulates _____
   and _____.

10. The cerebellum coordinates _____.
    It also helps to maintain _____
    and _____.

11. Pyramidal tracts carry impulses from the brain to
    the spinal cord to the _____.

12. Extrapyramidal tracts do not enter the
    _____.

13. A lack of oxygen is called _____.

14. Hypoglycemia causes _____,
    _____, _____,
    _____, and _____.

15. _____ is required for the pro-
    duction and use of glucose.

16. A thiamine deficiency can cause degeneration of
    the _____ and can lead to
    _____ syndrome.

17. Moderate CNS depression produces
    _____, _____,
    _____, and _____
    _____.

18. Severe CNS depression produces
    _____, loss of reflexes,
    _____, and _____.

19. Mild CNS stimulants produce _____,
    _____, and _____.

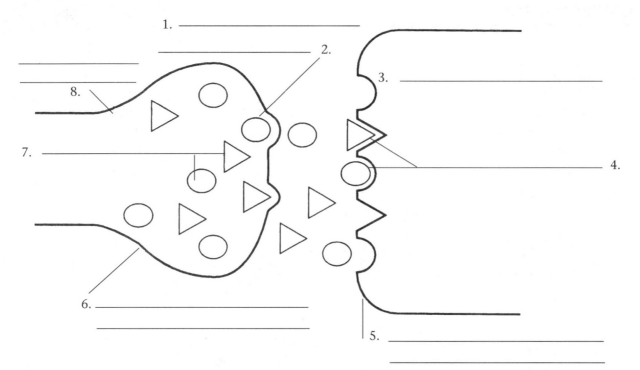

1. _____

2. _____

3. _____

4. _____

5. _____

6. _____

7. _____

8.

Figure 5-1

20. Moderate CNS stimulants produce

_____, _____,

_____, and _____.

21. Excessive CNS stimulation can cause

_____, _____,

and _____.

Neurotransmission, Part I

Neurotransmitter molecules, released by the presynaptic nerve, cross the synapse and bind with receptor proteins in the cell membrane of the postsynaptic nerve.

Fill in the blanks in Figure 5-1 with the terms below.

Receptor sites

Neurotransmitters

Presynaptic nerve terminal

Presynaptic nerve cell membrane

Postsynaptic nerve terminal

Synapse

Release site

Postsynaptic nerve cell membrane

Neurotransmission, Part II

Complete the following sentences.

1. Norepinephrine is an excitatory neurotransmitter that affects mood and motor activity after crossing the _____ from the postganglionic sympathetic nervous system neurons and binding to _____ in the postsynaptic nerve cell membrane of the nerves that supply blood vessels to the adrenal medulla.

2. Acetylcholine is an inhibitory neurotransmitter that exerts inhibitory effects on organs supplied by the vagus nerves by binding at

_____.

REVIEW QUESTIONS

1. Your client has had a CVA and he has short-term memory loss. Which part of his brain was affected by the CVA?
   a. Limbic system.
   b. Reticular formation network.
   c. Cerebral cortex.
   d. Cerebellum.

2. Glucose is required for
   a. adequate cerebral blood flow.
   b. cell metabolism.
   c. oxygen utilization.
   d. transference of nerve impulses.

3. Lack of dopamine causes Parkinson's disease, which is characterized by
   a. hyperactive reflexes and muscle spasms.
   b. slurred speech and memory loss.
   c. muscle weakness and dizziness.
   d. rigidity and increased muscle tone.

4. Thirst and appetite centers are located in the
   a. thalamus.
   b. cerebellum.
   c. medulla oblongata.
   d. hypothalamus.

5. Mild CNS depression can produce
   a. short attention span.
   b. decreased muscle tone.
   c. decreased perception of sensation.
   d. loss of reflexes.

6. The area of the brain responsible for temperature regulation is the
   a. limbic system.
   b. cerebellum.
   c. medulla oblongata.
   d. hypothalamus.

7. After surgery, Mr. S.'s respiratory rate falls to 10. Which portion of the brain helps to regulate respiration?
   a. Medulla oblongata.
   b. Limbic system.
   c. Hypothalamus.
   d. Cerebrum.

8. Severe hypoglycemia can cause
   a. degeneration of the myelin sheath.
   b. encephalopathy.
   c. seizures.
   d. hypotension.

9. After a tumor is removed from the cerebellum, the nurse needs to monitor
   a. muscular coordination.
   b. memory loss.
   c. respiratory depression.
   d. intake and output.

10. Excessive CNS stimulation can cause
    a. insomnia.
    b. excessive talking.
    c. nervousness.
    d. cardiac dysrhythmias.

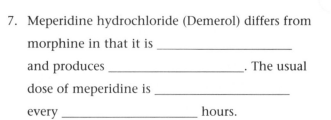

Narcotic Analgesics and Narcotic Antagonists

FILL IN THE BLANKS

Complete the following sentences.

1. CNS effects of narcotic analgesics include:

   a. _____

   b. _____

   c. _____

   d. _____

   e. _____

2. Narcotics affect the GI system by _____ and causing _____.

3. Morphine sulfate can be administered _____, _____, and _____.

4. Roxanol _____/ml and MS Contin _____ tab/sustained release have been developed for cancer patients with chronic pain.

5. Fentanyl (Duragesic) is administered by _____ and lasts _____.

6. Codeine is often given with _____ or _____.

7. Meperidine hydrochloride (Demerol) differs from morphine in that it is _____ and produces _____. The usual dose of meperidine is _____ every _____ hours.

8. Three examples of non-narcotic drugs used for moderate to severe pain are _____, _____, and _____.

9. A narcotic antagonist used to treat narcotic overdoses is _____.

10. Before administering pain medication you should _____.

11. Besides the administration of pain medications, other nursing measures that can be employed include _____, application of _____, and _____ techniques.

12. Three responses that a nurse must understand before administering pain medications are _____, _____, and _____.

13. The _____ route of administration is preferred when administering narcotics for acute pain because _____.

14. A _____ allows clients to self-administer pain medication.

15. The recommendation for narcotic use is _____ to 72 hours except for malignant disease.

16. _____ can be used with narcotic analgesics for the treatment of various types of colic because it reduces the spasms caused by narcotic analgesics.

17. Infants may respond to pain by

    _____, _____,

    or with _____.

18. Before administering narcotics the nurse should

    check the client's _____ rate.

19. After pain medication has been administered,

    the client should be instructed to not

    _____ or

    _____ without help.

20. _____ is used for clients with

    pulmonary edema because it causes

    _____, which _____

    venous return and _____ car-

    diac work.

21. Adverse reactions from pain medication include

    _____, _____,

    _____, _____,

    and constipation.

22. Persons taking pain medications should not

    drink _____.

WORD SCRAMBLE

Unscramble the words below, then circle them in the Word Find.

1. _____ yatnfeln
2. _____ edeiocin
3. _____ ormdeel
4. _____ dladdiiu
5. _____ pimorhen

6. _____ adtods
7. _____ ovardn
8. _____ nbinua
9. _____ craann
10. _____ inwtal

Word Find

```
N O T H S B H Y P O F T I L C L C E F G H H J N K
K A D R E N E R G I C E N B E T A Z O L O L A N E
C M R I A S S A N L L X Q K E Z S V C D N C A T V
X Y Z T I P L D N E D R O N O N I R L A R N V R R
H L P O D I L A U D I D I C A Y Y O D A V V P P J
F N V A N L I C B R E E K X F H T G N A E S O S B
R I L U A A C A I D D U K L O E E U U E T O R R P
X T O S H R F R N O H A Z Y P X D K B B L K A O T
L R N A Y J R E C L N O S T Y H P E A N B E R E C
V A S G O N I Q P F E N T A N Y L K I S N L O K C
X T K X T G A A N G N P A P E C O R N I U O U S A
K J K X C Z A B T N T A D P V C D T E G F G X H O
V A S D I P I O C P R A O Z O I N J K A J K L D N
O N A E S O R P T I O N L W N C I N U C N C I V O
P T O M I I A N G I N Y B W I X K U N L S I N E T
A Z A E Y B I D L E S X F N I N S V D F H I A N I
R S C R F X Z Y N G R H V T G N J N A A E Z H T L
G E M O R P H I N E V K O N M H C H L O R Z I D E
Y N O L G D B P Q E R R O T V S P Q Y L O V B P C
L W I E F I C D L S N E V H O W G Y O Z A J O W D
F D O M R G G L I I S T P R O T E R E N E R Z N X
N C O E U M A D I N S F T P T M I G J F U W T C Y
E F D D Q C N Q N T A T D Y M N S J Z E B G O G C
```

REVIEW QUESTIONS

1. Which of the following assessments is attributable to the administration of narcotics?
   a. Tachycardia.
   b. Hypertension.
   c. Hyperactive bowel sounds.
   d. Pupillary constriction.

2. When you administer morphine, it is important to assess for
   a. respiratory depression.
   b. absent bowel sounds.
   c. bradycardia.
   d. decreased urinary output.

3. An example of a narcotic analgesic used for moderate pain is
   a. oxymorphone hydrochloride (Numorphan).
   b. codeine sulfate.
   c. morphine sulfate (Roxanol).
   d. butorphanol tartrate (Stadol).

4. A common side effect of the administration of opiates is
   a. constipation.
   b. bradycardia.
   c. dry mouth.
   d. blurred vision.

5. A physician during World War II ran out of pain medication for his men who had been injured in battle, so he administered normal saline and the men were relieved of their pain. This is an example of
   a. pain threshold.
   b. pain perception.
   c. behavioral response.
   d. placebo response.

6. The drug of choice for pain relief for end-stage cancer patients is
   a. morphine sulfate (Roxanol).
   b. propoxyphene (Darvon).
   c. codeine sulfate.
   d. meperidine hydrochloride (Demerol).

7. Which of the following statements by Mr. C. leads you to believe that he understands the preoperative teaching you have done?
   a. "I will ask for medication every 4 hours whether I need it or not."
   b. "I will take the pain medication so that I will be able to turn, cough, and take a deep breath."
   c. "I will avoid taking the pain medication because it will impair my ability to ambulate and impede my recovery."
   d. "No matter how bad the pain gets, I am not to ask for medication before 4 hours."

8. Pain relieving substances produced by the body include
   a. opioids.
   b. histamine.
   c. bradykinins.
   d. endorphins.

9. Which of the following medications, if administered concurrently with morphine, may produce hypotension?
   a. Antihistamines.
   b. Antidiabetic agents.
   c. Thyroid preparations.
   d. Diuretics.

10. The physician has ordered a PCA (patient controlled analgesia) pump or infusion for Mrs. J. after her abdominal surgery to
    a. relieve the nursing staff of q4h administration of pain medication.
    b. eliminate the administration of IV medications.
    c. provide small amounts of pain medication at regular intervals throughout the day.
    d. reduce the amount of pain medication used.

CRITICAL THINKING CASE STUDY

M.G., a 29-year-old, had a simple mastectomy 3 days ago. She has been receiving meperidine hydrochloride (Demerol) IM every 4 hours for pain since returning from surgery. You medicate her with two Tylenol #3 at 10:30 A.M. Before you help her out of bed she states, "The Demerol makes me feel so much better. I don't think this medication is going to work."

1. How you would respond to her statement?

2. Describe the adverse effects you are assessing for.

While you are at lunch, M.G. requests Demerol and one of your colleagues administers it.

3. Discuss what you would do when you return from lunch and find out M.G. has been medicated.

7

Analgesic-, Antipyretic-, Anti-inflammatory and Related Drugs

F. Naproxen (Naprosyn).

G. Advil.

H. Allopurinol (Zyloprim).

I. Prostaglandins.

J. Fever.

K. Headache.

MATCHING EXERCISE

Terms and Concepts

Match the concept with the term for it.

1. _____ Toxic doses of this drug can cause liver necrosis.

2. _____ This drug has antiplatelet properties.

3. _____ The normal body response to tissue damage.

4. _____ Substances found in body tissue that help regulate cell function.

5. _____ A drug used in the treatment of gout.

6. _____ A drug used only for the treatment of migraine headaches.

7. _____ An ibuprofen drug available without a prescription.

8. _____ A classic sign of an aspirin overdose.

9. _____ A NSAID effective in the treatment of juvenile arthritis.

10. _____ May be caused by dehydration, infectious process and brain injury.

A. Inflammation.

B. Ergotamine tartrate (Ergomar).

C. Ringing in the ears.

D. Acetaminophen (Tylenol).

E. Acetylsalicylic acid (ASA).

TRUE OR FALSE

1. _____ Gangrene of the extremities has occurred after the administration of ergotamine tartrate (Ergomar).

2. _____ Therapeutic effects from ergot preparations are usually evident within an hour after the drug is administered.

3. _____ When diuretics are administered with allopurinol (Zyloprim), the effect of allopurinol (Zyloprim) is increased.

4. _____ Persons taking indomethacin (Indocin) need to be assessed for confusion and depression.

5. _____ Clients receiving methysergide maleate (Sansert) should be examined frequently for pulmonary fibrosis and fibrotic thickening of cardiac valves and arteries.

6. _____ Diflunisal (Dolobid) is equal or superior to ASA for arthritis pain.

7. _____ Ketoprofen (Orudis) is better tolerated than ASA but can still cause many of the adverse effects associated with ASA.

8. _____ No anti-inflammatory/analgesic medication can be administered parenterally.

REVIEW QUESTIONS

1. A 29-year-old male is admitted with chronic ergot poisoning. You should be assessing him for

   a. neurotoxicity.

   b. renal failure.

   c. hepatotoxicity.

   d. circulatory impairment.

2. Which of the following medications, if administered concurrently with sulfinpyrazone (Anturane), will decrease its effects?

   a. Aspirin.

   b. Acetaminophen (Tylenol).

   c. Antidiabetic agents.

   d. Maalox.

3. A client taking an ergot preparation for a migraine headache should be told to report

   a. nausea and vomiting.

   b. sore throat and fever.

   c. skin rash or upset stomach.

   d. numbness or tingling of the extremities.

4. Which of the following statements by your client leads you to believe that she has understood the teaching that you have done about relief of migraine headaches?

   a. "I will take the medication only after I have tried other remedies."

   b. "After taking the medication, I should get relief of headache pain within 5–10 minutes."

   c. "After I take the medication, I will lie down in a quiet dark room."

   d. "If I think there is a possibility that I might get a headache, I will take the medication."

5. The drug used in the treatment of gout that lowers uric acid levels is

   a. ibuprofen (Motrin).

   b. allopurinol (Zyloprim).

   c. hydroxychloroquine (Plaquenil).

   d. cyclophosphamide (Cytoxan).

6. Your client is started on indomethacin (Indocin). Which of the following statements leads you to believe that he understands the adverse effects of this medication?

   a. "If I have difficulty with balance or walking, I will contact my physician."

   b. "I will call my physician if I experience headaches."

   c. "I may have a low grade fever late in the afternoon."

   d. "I can anticipate diarrhea so I will avoid foods high in roughage."

7. Which of the following medications, if administered concurrently with aspirin, will increase its effects?

   a. Ascorbic acid (vitamin C).

   b. Misoprostol (Cytotec).

   c. Sodium bicarbonate.

   d. Thiazide diuretics.

8. Your client is started on cyclophosphamide (Cytoxan). Which of the following lab values should be assessed on a regular basis?

   a. Hematocrit.

   b. WBC.

   c. Uric acid levels.

   d. Serum glucose.

9. Mr. B. is admitted with visual changes, drowsiness, hearing difficulty, confusion, and hyperventilation. These symptoms may be attributable to

   a. acute acetaminophen (Tylenol) poisoning.

   b. salicylate intoxication.

   c. acute ergot poisoning.

   d. hyperuricemia.

10. Your client has started taking aspirin for the pain and stiffness associated with arthritis. When can he or she expect to see improvement of symptoms?

    a. 3–4 hours.

    b. 6–12 hours.

    c. 24–48 hours.

    d. 48–72 hours.

CRITICAL THINKING CASE STUDY

Mr. J., a 55-year-old teacher, has been prescribed sulindac (Clinoril) for rheumatoid arthritis that has been unresponsive to other drugs. In reviewing Mr. J.'s record, you find that he has a history of psychosis, diabetes, hypertension, and anemia.

1. Identify what in the client's history should be discussed with the physician before sulindac (Clinoril) is started and why.

2. Identify the periodic assessments that will be planned for this client.

Mr. J. is experiencing severe pain. His physician prescribes ketorolac (Toradol).

4. Describe how you will explain the rationale for the change in medication to the client.

3. Discuss the teaching you will do with this client.

8

Antianxiety and Sedative-Hypnotic Drugs

FILL IN THE BLANKS

1. When anxiety is_____, it impairs the ability to function.

2. The classification of anxiety disorder includes _____, _____, _____, _____, _____, and _____.

3. REM (_____) sleep is thought to be _____.

4. Insomnia may be caused by _____, _____, _____, _____, and _____.

5. _____, _____, and other drugs are used to treat anxiety and insomnia.

6. Barbiturates stimulate _____ to produce large amounts of drug metabolizing enzymes; this is referred to as _____.

7. Benzodiazepines can cause _____ and _____ dependence.

8. Benzodiazepines are _____ soluble and bind to _____.

9. Some benzodiazepines have a _____ half-life and require _____ days to reach a steady state.

10. Buspirone (_____) causes less _____ and does not cause _____ or _____ dependence but lacks the _____ and _____ effects of benzodiazepines.

11. Hydroxyzine (_____) has _____ and _____ properties.

12. _____, the oldest sedative hypnotic is _____, effective, and _____, but _____ develops quickly.

13. Antihistamines such as _____ (_____) also cause drowsiness.

14. Benzodiazepines are used as _____, _____, and _____ agents. They are also used for preoperative sedation and to prevent _____ and _____ in acute alcohol withdrawal.

15. Benzodiazepines are contraindicated in _____, _____, and _____ and for clients with a history of _____.

16. Clinical manifestations of benzodiazepine withdrawal syndrome include _____, _____, _____, _____, _____, _____, _____, and _____. More serious manifestations include _____, _____, _____, _____, and _____.

17. _____ (_____)

    is an antidote for benzodiazepines.

18. In the presence of liver disease, the benzodi-

    azepines of choice are _____

    (_____) and _____

    (_____).

NURSING DIAGNOSIS

Mrs. J has recently been diagnosed with ALS. She is
extremely anxious and her physician has placed her
on antianxiety medication. Identify three possible
nursing diagnoses, pertinent assessment data, and
nursing interventions.

1. Nursing Diagnosis:

    Assessment Data:

    Nursing Interventions:

2. Nursing Diagnosis:

    Assessment Data:

    Nursing Interventions:

3. Nursing Diagnosis:

    Assessment Data:

    Nursing Interventions:

DEFINITION

Define the following term.

1. Anxiety

    _____

REVIEW QUESTIONS

1. Ms. A has been using alprazolam (Xanax) for 1
   week for insomnia. She states that she is sleeping
   at night but does not feel rested. This is probably
   due to a reduction in
   a. Stage I sleep.
   b. Stage II sleep.
   c. Stage III sleep.
   d. REM sleep.

2. The following instructions should be given to
   clients who are to receive alprazolam (Xanax):
   a. If you experience drowsiness, discontinue the
      medication.
   b. Avoid alcohol.
   c. If you are unable to sleep at night, take 1½
      tablets.
   d. Take the medication as you need it for anxi-
      ety.

3. Abruptly stopping alprazolam (Xanax) can result
   in
   a. seizures.
   b. headaches.
   c. dermatitis.
   d. rebound tachycardia.

4. You should assess a client receiving benzodiazepines for
   a. reduced albumin.
   b. elevated creatinine.
   c. elevated bilirubin.
   d. reduced platelets.

5. When a benzodiazepine is administered preoperatively for sleep, you should instruct the client
   that he or she can anticipate the desired effect
   within
   a. 15 minutes.
   b. 90 minutes.
   c. 45 minutes.
   d. 60 minutes.

6. A sedative that is also used as a skeletal muscle relaxant is
   a. alprazolam (Xanax).
   b. diazepam (Valium).
   c. midazolam (Versed).
   d. lorazepam (Ativan).

7. Benzodiazepines
   a. potentiate effects of other CNS depressants.
   b. produce little dependence when given as recommended.
   c. are associated with gastritis when given with caffeine.
   d. are absorbed slowly when given orally.

8. Chlordiazepoxide (Librium)
   a. peaks rapidly when administered intramuscularly.
   b. has no cumulative effects.
   c. is commonly used for treating alcohol withdrawal.
   d. is used for situational anxiety.

9. The benzodiazepine associated with memory impairment is
   a. alprazolam (Xanax).
   b. diazepam (Valium).
   c. midazolam (Versed).
   d. lorazepam (Ativan).

10. Antianxiety medications
    a. only need to be administered for 2 weeks.
    b. eliminate all feelings of distress.
    c. aid in symptomatic relief.
    d. produce a cure for anxiety reactions.

9

Antipsychotic Drugs

FILL IN THE BLANKS

Complete the following sentences.

1. _____ is a severe mental disorder characterized by disorganized and often bizarre thinking.

2. _____ are perceptions of people or objects that are not present.

3. _____ are false beliefs that persist in the absence of evidence.

4. Symptoms of _____ usually begin in adolescence or early adulthood.

5. _____ is the most common chronic psychosis.

6. The prototypical group of antipsychotic drugs is _____.

7. Phenothiazine exerts many pharmacologic effects, including _____, _____, _____, _____, and _____.

8. Antipsychotic drugs decrease the effects of _____.

9. Antipsychotic drugs decrease hyperarousal, which includes symptoms of

   _____, _____, _____, _____, _____/_____ behavior, _____, and delusions.

10. Clinical indications for the use of antipsychotics that are not associated with psychiatric illness include treatment of _____, _____, and intractable hiccups.

11. Promethazine (_____) is used for its _____, _____, and _____ effects.

12. Chlorprothixene (_____) and thiothixene (_____) are used for their _____ effects.

13. Haloperidol (_____) produces a _____ incidence of _____ and _____ and a _____ incidence of _____.

14. Haldol is also used in _____, _____, and _____.

15. Extrapyramidal effects produced by some antipsychotic medications include

    _____, _____, _____, and _____.

16. Loxapine (_____) and clozapine (_____) are used for the treatment of schizophrenia. Clozapine has a high risk of _____ and other adverse effects, including _____, _____, and ECG changes.

17. Pimozide (Orap) is used for the treatment of _____. Serious adverse effects include _____, _____, and _____.

18. Goals of treatment with antipsychotic drugs are to _____, _____, and _____.

19. Some clients who do not respond well to one type of antipsychotic drug may _____. If a substitution of a new drug is necessary, the old drug should be decreased while substituting _____ doses of the new drug.

20. Clients who are unable or unwilling to take daily doses of antipsychotic drugs may be given _____ of _____.

21. The best time to administer antipsychotic drugs is _____ daily within _____ of bedtime.

22. Liquid concentrates should be mixed with _____ of _____ or _____.

23. Antiadrenergic effects include _____, _____, _____, _____, and _____.

24. Anticholinergic effects include _____, dental _____, _____, _____, _____, and _____.

25. Endocrine effects include _____, _____, _____ in males, and _____.

CAUTION OR CONTRAINDICATION

*Place **ca** in front of the conditions for which antipsychotic medications should be used with **caution** and **ci** in front of the conditions for which the use of antipsychotics is **contraindicated**.*

1. _____ Liver damage.

2. _____ Coronary artery disease.

3. _____ CVA.

4. _____ Seizure disorders.

5. _____ Diabetes mellitus.

6. _____ Parkinson's disease.

7. _____ Glaucoma.

8. _____ Peptic ulcer disease.

9. _____ Bone marrow depression.

10. _____ Hypertension.

11. _____ Chronic respiratory disorders.

12. _____ Severe depressive states.

13. _____ Coma.

WORD SCRAMBLE

Fill in the trade name next to the generic name, then circle the trade name in the word find.

1. acetophenazine _____

2. thioridazine _____

3. prochlorperazine _____

4. fluphenazine hydrochloride

   _____

5. chlorpromazine _____

6. perphenazine _____

7. promazine _____

8. trifluoperazine _____

9. molindone _____

10. pimozide _____

11. clozapine _____

12. haloperidol _____

13. chlorprothixene _____

14. thiothixene _____

15. loxapine _____

Word Find

```
T A L E F D F D Q C N Q N S P A R I N E T X A T W
A N C O E K N U M O A R D I Q N B P N T P T M I H
R G P T M T M I G J F U W T C Y I I D E O M R G K
A G G L I I S T M N P K R O T E Z R E N R E Z N X
C L L W I N E F I C D E L S N A X U O W Y O Z A R
T Y O N R D G S D B P W B R P R O T V S P Q V Y L
A V G E M A A O R H P H I M E V K O F N M H T M I
N Z R B T L C L O I X M O B A N I X E U Z Y R N G
R H V T G H F J J N A C L O Z A R I L E A Z I H O
A T L Y A Z O Y B I D L E S P X T F N D N S L S V
D F H I M D F R U T P T O R T I D S H L B Z A T E
X O N A B Q S O A R P P T I U O N D C O W N F C I
R U C N K I V O V Z A S H Q O I P C P X R A O L Z
F K J K Z X C Z A M I B T A N D A O A I P V N C D
G C D T X E C F J G E N F G L X H O L T E B T M O
C D T I P B Q T U D H L E R A D P D A A P X D A T
P L A A W S M A X V T G L A A G O N P N A P E C N
O R R N I U O Q U S P U S A V A S L G E O N E I Q
P O F E J N T A N Y L K I R S B N C L K I S N L
O K C P L V R N A I A Y J R E I C L N O S W T Y H
P E A R B S E R E V C X T S T E L A Z I N E T O S
P R O L I X I N X A A S O N I Q U G P E N T A N Y
L K I S N G L O O K L N R N A Y J R E C L I N O S
T Y H P E A M B E R E C E P X T O S H R F R N O H
H M A Z Y P X D R M B B L K A O T R I L U A A C B
```

REVIEW QUESTIONS

1. Six weeks after starting chlorpromazine (Thorazine), your client complains of difficulty chewing and swallowing. You should

   a. crush Mrs. P.'s medications.

   b. place Mrs. P. on a full liquid diet.

   c. puree all Mrs. P.'s food.

   d. contact the physician.

2. Your client is taking chlorpromazine (Thorazine). The following symptom should be reported to the physician immediately:

   a. Loss of appetite.

   b. Dry mouth.

   c. Diarrhea.

   d. Sore throat.

3. Mrs. T.'s husband is dying of cancer, and he is psychotic and extremely agitated. His physician orders haloperidol (Haldol) 2 mg q2h PRN until his symptoms are controlled. Mrs. T. asks you when Mr. T.'s symptoms will be controlled. Your *best* response would be the following:

   a. It will take three or four doses before we see any results.

   b. He should begin to calm down within the hour.

   c. The symptoms are usually controlled within 72 hours.

   d. If we medicate him every 2 hours around the clock, he will be calm by tomorrow morning.

4. Your client is presently taking propranolol (Inderal). Her physician starts her on perphenazine (Trilafon) for psychosis. You know that

   a. the dosage of Trilafon may need to be increased because she is using Inderal.

   b. the dosage of Trilafon may need to be decreased because she is using Inderal.

   c. the dosage of Inderal may need to be increased because Trilafon was added.

   d. no change in dosage needs to be made.

5. M.J. is admitted for a psychotic episode. He attempts to bite an orderly while he is being restrained. When you administer IM chlorpromazine (Thorazine) to M.J. you should

   a. question him about his feelings.

   b. demonstrate a calm, firm manner.

   c. ask him where he would like the injection.

   d. wait for him to calm down.

6. Which of these statements by your client, who has been started on perphenazine (Trilafon), indicates that she understands the instructions you have given her?

   a. "I will see my dentist every six months and brush my teeth frequently."

   b. "I will only go outside at night."

   c. "I will lie down for an hour after each dose of the medication."

   d. "I will take antacids with my medication."

7. When doing discharge teaching with your client who is taking thioridazine (Mellaril), which of the following instructions is appropriate?

   a. "You need to see the doctor weekly to have a white blood cell count done."

   b. "Use a sunscreen and wear protective clothing when out in the sun."

   c. "A diet high in fiber with a good fluid intake will help you maintain normal bowel habits."

   d. "Discontinue the medication if you are drowsy or dizzy."

8. Mr. H., who is taking antipsychotic medication, starts smacking his lips, protruding his tongue, and engaging in facial grimacing. Based on these findings, the nurse should suspect

   a. increased psychosis.

   b. dystonia.

   c. tardive dyskinesia.

   d. Parkinsonism.

9. After assessing Mrs. J., who has just been admitted to your unit, you obtain the following data: BP 160/70, pulse 98, respiration 26, temperature 96.2°. Which one of these findings could be attributed to the use of antipsychotic medications?

   a. Blood pressure.

   b. Pulse.

   c. Respiration.

   d. Temperature.

10. The best time to administer oral antipsychotic drugs that are administered once a day is

   a. upon awakening.

   b. with breakfast.

   c. before dinner.

   d. 1–2 hours before bedtime.

CRITICAL THINKING CASE STUDY

Mr. P., an 89-year-old, is admitted from home with a diagnosis of psychosis. He is agitated and combative. The following laboratory tests were ordered: SGOT/AST, WBC, Na$^+$, K$^+$, Cl$^-$, glucose.

1. Identify medical conditions in which the use of antipsychotic medications would be contraindicated.

Mr. J. is started on fluphenazine hydrochloride (Prolixin) IM.

2. Determine what an appropriate dose for Mr. P. would be and discuss how you came to the conclusion.

3. Discuss why this medication was chosen.

Mr. P.'s daughter is very concerned about him and asks when she can expect to see improvement in his condition.

4. Discuss your response to Mr. P.'s daughter.

Four days after admission, Mr. P.'s daughter is very upset because he is sleeping all the time.

5. Explain to Mr. P.'s daughter what she can expect.

One month after admission, Mr. P. develops compulsive involuntary restless movements. Mr. P.'s daughter questions whether the psychosis has returned.

6. Describe your response to Mr. P.'s daughter.

Mr. P.'s daughter plans on taking him home to live with her.

7. Discuss what instructions she should be given.

10

Antidepressants

FILL IN THE BLANKS

Complete the following sentences.

1. Symptoms of depression include

   a. _____

   b. _____

   c. _____

   d. _____

   e. _____

   f. _____

   g. _____

   h. _____

   i. _____

   j. _____

   k. _____

2. Secondary depression may be precipitated by

   _____, _____,

   and _____.

3. Tricyclic antidepressants produce

   _____, _____,

   and cardiac dysrhythmias.

4. Amitriptyline (_____) and

   imipramine (Tofranil) are commonly used

   _____.

5. Monoamine oxidase inhibitors may interact with

   _____ and _____

   to produce _____.

6. Foods that interact with MAO inhibitors are

   those containing _____.

7. Identify eight commonly eaten foods that are
   high in tyramine.

   a. _____

   b. _____

   c. _____

   d. _____

   e. _____

   f. _____

   g. _____

   h. _____

8. Fluoxetine (_____), a serotonin

   reuptake inhibitor, can produce common adverse

   effects, which include _____,

   _____, _____,

   and _____.

9. Lithium carbonate (_____) is

   used for clients with _____.

10. _____ is a prerequisite for lithi-

    um therapy.

11. Deviations in serum _____

    affect lithium levels.

12. TCAs and MAOs are given for _____.

13. Lithium may be given for _____.

14. A therapeutic effect from TCAs is expected in

    _____ weeks.

15. For most clients the therapeutic serum level for

    lithium is _____ mEq/liter.

16. It takes _____ weeks before the

    therapeutic effects from MAOs are seen.

17. Commonly seen adverse effects from TCAs when treatment is initiated include _____, _____, _____, _____, _____, _____, _____, and _____ sweating.

18. Adverse effects seen with higher drug levels of lithium include _____, _____, _____, _____, _____, _____, _____, _____, and _____.

SENTENCE CORRECTION

Circle the word that makes the sentence incorrect and place the correct word in the space provided. Example: <u>contraindicated</u> *Antidepressants are (<u>commonly used</u>) for clients with schizophrenia.*

1. _____ An adverse effect of antidepressants that is useful in treating enuresis is insomnia.

2. _____ Furosemide (Lasix) should not be administered with MAO inhibitors because a hypertensive crisis could occur.

3. _____ A deficiency of potassium increases the risk of lithium toxicity.

4. _____ Fluoxetine (Prozac) needs to be administered b.i.d.

5. _____ Blurred vision should be reported to the physician for persons taking MAO inhibitors.

6. _____ Adequate hepatic function is a prerequisite for lithium therapy.

7. _____ Depression results from a deficiency of dopamine and acetylcholine.

8. _____ Tricyclic antidepressants produce a relatively high incidence of cardiac failure.

9. _____ Gastric lavage is the preferred treatment for severe lithium overdose.

10. _____ Caffeine decreases the effects of tricyclic antidepressants.

11. _____ If therapeutic effects from TCAs are not seen in 8 weeks, the medication should be discontinued.

12. _____ Lithium is used to control severe depression.

13. _____ Diazepam (Valium) is used to reverse anticholinergic effects of TCAs.

14. _____ Serum lithium levels should be drawn every 6 months.

15. _____ TCAs are not recommended for persons under the age of 18 except for treatment of enuresis; then they may be used in children over age 12.

CRITICAL THINKING CASE STUDY

Mrs. J. is admitted to your unit with a diagnosis of depression.

1. Discuss how the diagnosis of depression is made.

Mrs. J. has a history of diabetes, gout, COPD, and allergies to pollen and animal dander.

2. Identify which of Mrs. J.'s illnesses need to be considered before antidepressants are prescribed.

The physician starts Mrs. J. on fluoxetine (Prozac).

3. Identify appropriate goals for Mr. J.

4. Specify the instruction Mrs. J. should be given before going home.

Mrs. J. returns to the clinic 3 weeks after starting antidepressant therapy complaining of anxiety and insomnia. Mrs. J. states that she is feeling worse and does not want to continue the medication.

5. Identify the assessments you will do.

6. Discuss how you will deal with Mrs. J.'s unwillingness to continue the medication.

REVIEW QUESTIONS

1. Which of the following nursing actions would take priority when caring for Mr. J., who is taking lithium?

   a. Monitor peripheral pulses.

   b. Provide a diet high in potassium.

   c. Provide a stimulating environment.

   d. Monitor fluid and electrolyte intake.

2. Foods that should be eliminated from the diet when a person is taking MAO inhibitors include

   a. oranges.

   b. chicken.

   c. eggs.

   d. cheese.

3. A client is admitted with a diagnosis of overdose of bupropion (Wellbutrin). Which of the following nursing diagnoses would be a priority?

   a. Potential for injury related to seizure activity.

   b. Knowledge deficit related to effects and usage of antidepressant.

   c. Sleep pattern disturbances related to depression.

   d. Alteration in thought process related to confusion.

4. Mr. J. is diagnosed with bipolar affective disorder and is to be started on lithium. He is taking aspirin, digoxin (Lanoxin), insulin, and furosemide (Lasix). Which of these medications must you make the physician aware of before you start the lithium?

   a. Aspirin.

   b. Digoxin (Lanoxin).

   c. Insulin.

   d. Furosemide (Lasix).

5. Which of the following medications, if administered concurrently with MAO inhibitors, will increase their effect?

   a. Hydrochlorothiazide (Oretic).

   b. Sodium bicarbonate.

   c. Theophylline.

   d. Meperidine (Demerol).

6. The nurse should assess the client who is taking lithium for symptoms of toxicity, which include

   a. bradycardia, hypotension, and apnea.

   b. blurred vision and polydipsia.

   c. fever and rash of the head and neck.

   d. tremors, oliguria, and confusion.

7. Which of the following statements by the client leads you to believe that he has understood the teaching that you have done regarding tricyclic antidepressants?

   a. "It is common to experience diarrhea. I will increase the fiber in my diet."

   b. "I may feel drowsy for a few weeks after the medication is started."

   c. "Nausea and vomiting are common in the first few weeks. I will eat small, frequent meals."

   d. "Skin rashes are common occurrences. I will stay out of the sun."

8. A lithium level is drawn, and it is 2.6 mEq/liter. You know that this level is

   a. below the therapeutic range.

   b. within the therapeutic range.

   c. slightly above the therapeutic range.

   d. indicative of toxicity.

9. When phenelzine (Nardil) is initiated, the nurse should assess the client for

   a. ataxia.

   b. hypotension.

   c. diarrhea.

   d. hyperglycemia.

10. A client who started taking lithium 2 days ago developed hand tremors. The best nursing action in this instance would be to

    a. administer propranolol (Inderal) to control the tremors.

    b. hold the lithium until the tremors subside.

    c. assure him that this is common and usually subsides within a few weeks.

    d. contact the physician immediately; stay with the client and have him remain in bed.

11

Anticonvulsants

FILL IN THE BLANKS

Complete the following sentences.

1. A seizure is a _____

   _____

2. A convulsion is a _____

   _____

3. Epilepsy is a _____

   _____

4. Epilepsy is diagnosed with an _____.

5. When epilepsy begins in infancy, it is caused by

   _____, _____,

   or _____.

6. Status epilepticus can be induced as a result of
   overdose of the following drugs:

   _____, _____,

   _____, and others.

7. A therapeutic Dilantin level is _____/ml.

8. Diazepam (_____) is used to

   terminate _____.

9. _____ (Tegretol) is used for

   clients with _____,

   _____, and _____

   seizures. Carbamazepine is also used to treat

   facial pain associated with _____.

10. The seven following things may produce seizures
    in people who have not had a previous history
    of seizures: _____,

    _____, _____,

    hypoxia, hypoglycemia, _____,

    and withdrawal from CNS depressants.

11. For most clients, convulsant therapy is

    _____.

12. Discontinuing or changing antiseizure drugs

    must be done over _____.

13. If phenytoin (Dilantin) is given intravenously,
    the intravenous line must be flushed before and

    after with _____, because if the

    phenytoin (Dilantin) mixes with a dextrose solu-

    tion it will _____.

14. _____ is the anticonvulsant of

    choice for absence seizures.

15. Many anticonvulsants decrease levels of

    _____, which can lead to mega-

    loblastic anemia.

TRUE OR FALSE

1. _____ A toxic level of lidocaine can produce
   seizures.

2. _____ During a seizure, a spoon should be
   inserted between the teeth to protect the
   tongue.

3. _____ Tonic–clonic seizures can result in
   agnosia, which lasts 3–4 hours after the
   seizure is over.

4. _____ Most anticonvulsant drugs have the
   potential for causing blood, liver, and kidney disorders.

5. _____ Oral anticonvulsants should be administered on an empty stomach.

6. _____ Alcohol increases the effect of phenytoin
   (Dilantin).

7. _____ Weight gain is common with persons taking anticonvulsant drugs.

CROSSWORD PUZZLE

Across

2. A tolerance to this drug can occur with long-term use.

4. A benzodiazepine used for acute alcohol withdrawal and to manage partial seizures.

5. The drug of choice for treating status epilepticus.

9. An anticonvulsant that is often used in conjunction with Dilantin.

Down

1. A type of seizure characterized by spasmodic reactions.

3. May cause life-threatening blood dyscrasia.

6. The initial drug of choice in adults who are experiencing tonic–clonic seizures.

7. Used to treat absence and mixed seizures.

8. A brain disorder that causes seizures.

10. Used to terminate acute seizures.

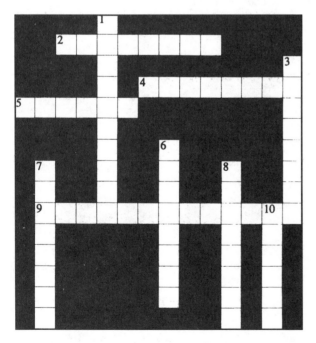

REVIEW QUESTIONS

1. The most important nursing diagnosis for a newly admitted client with a seizure disorder is
   a. risk for injury.
   b. ineffective coping.
   c. knowledge deficit.
   d. self-care deficit.

2. The drug of choice for treating generalized seizures in infants is
   a. phenobarbital.
   b. clonazepam (Klonopin).
   c. phenytoin (Dilantin).
   d. diazepam (Valium).

3. A therapeutic phenobarbital level is
   a. 2–7 µg/ml.
   b. 10–25 µg/ml.
   c. 25–50 µg/ml.
   d. 40–50 µg/ml.

4. Which of the following drugs is most effective for treating acute alcohol withdrawal?
   a. Carbamazepine (Tegretol).
   b. Clonazepam (Klonopin).
   c. Clorazepate (Tranxene).
   d. Ethosuximide (Zarontin).

5. The dosage of phenytoin (Dilantin) may need to be adjusted if your client is taking
   a. beta blockers.
   b. anticholinergics.
   c. oral contraceptives.
   d. calcium channel blockers.

6. Persons taking valproic acid (Depakene) must be observed for
   a. abnormal liver function.
   b. weight gain.
   c. night blindness.
   d. abnormal blood glucose levels.

7. Mr. J. is in ICU after open heart surgery. He is receiving theophylline, digoxin, Nipride, and nitroglycerin. Mr. J. experiences a seizure. A toxic effect from which of the drugs that he is receiving could have produced the seizure?
   a. Theophylline.
   b. Nipride.
   c. Digoxin.
   d. Nitroglycerin.

8. M. is admitted to the ER and begins to have rapid rhythmic and symmetric jerking movements of her body. You would document this as a

   a. partial seizure.

   b. focal seizure.

   c. petit mal seizure.

   d. major motor seizure.

9. When administering a loading dose of phenytoin (Dilantin), the nurse should observe the client closely for

   a. hypertension.

   b. respiratory depression.

   c. hypotension.

   d. decreased level of consciousness.

10. Your client is receiving 100 mg of phenytoin (Dilantin) b.i.d. His Dilantin level is 30 μg/ml. You would expect to

    a. administer the dosage as ordered.

    b. decrease the daily dosage.

    c. hold the drug until further orders.

    d. increase the daily dosage.

CRITICAL THINKING CASE STUDY

C.M., a 16-year-old girl, has been admitted to your unit with a head injury. She has been having intermittent seizures since her hospitalization 24 hours ago. (Learners may need to use additional sources to answer these questions.)

1. Describe what you will do if C.M. has another seizure.

The physician prescribes phenytoin (Dilantin) 100 mg b.i.d. and phenobarbital 20 mg b.i.d. for C.M.

2. Discuss why her physician ordered two anticonvulsants.

After 2 days C.M. develops a rash all over her body.

3. Identify your nursing actions in response to C.M.'s rash.

C.M. asks you if she will have to take the medication the rest of her life.

4. Describe your response.

C.M. is discharged on primidone (Mysoline).

5. Describe the teaching that you will do before discharge.

12

Antiparkinson Drugs

FILL IN THE BLANKS

Complete the following sentences.

1. Parkinson's disease is a _____, _____, _____ disorder of the CNS characterized by _____, _____, and _____.

2. People with Parkinson's disease have a decrease in _____ and an increase in _____.

3. Dopaminergic drugs that exert beneficial effects in Parkinson's disease are _____ (Dopar), carbidopa (_____), amantadine (_____), and bromocriptine (_____).

4. Amantadine (_____) increases _____.

5. Bromocriptine (Parlodel) stimulates _____.

6. Anticholinergic drugs are contraindicated in clients with _____, _____, _____, urinary bladder _____, and _____.

7. Levodopa (Larodopa) (Dopar) is the _____ drug available for the treatment of Parkinson's disease.

8. With long-term use of levodopa (Dopar), clients experience _____ of parkinsonism symptoms.

9. A levodopa–carbidopa combination product is _____, which allows more levodopa to reach the _____.

10. Amantadine (_____) relieves parkinsonism symptoms in _____ days, but loses its effectiveness in 6–8 weeks of continuous administration.

11. Bromocriptine (Parlodel) may _____ of levodopa and reduce the _____.

12. Levodopa is the drug of choice when _____ and _____ are the prominent symptoms.

TRUE OR FALSE

1. _____ Levodopa (Dopar) and bromocriptine (Parlodel) should be given on an empty stomach.

2. _____ Anticholinergic drugs produce atropine-line effects.

3. _____ Dyskinesia is a side effect of levodopa and results in involuntary movements of the tongue, mouth, face, or whole body.

4. _____ Persons taking levodopa should be observed for bradycardia.

5. _____ Bromocriptine (Parlodel) can produce a patchy blue discoloration on skin on the legs called livedo reticularis.

6. _____ Persons taking levodopa need to increase their intake of protein and vitamin B6.

REVIEW QUESTIONS

1. Your client is to go home on levodopa (Dopar). Which of the following statements leads you to believe that he has understood the teaching that you have done?
   a. "I will limit my fluid intake to 1500 ml a day."
   b. "I will avoid yellow vegetables."
   c. "I will increase the fiber in my diet."
   d. "I will limit my intake of alcohol and protein."

2. Levodopa is contraindicated for use in persons who have
   a. migraine headaches.
   b. peptic ulcer disease.
   c. thyroid disease.
   d. glaucoma.

3. Amantadine hydrochloride (Symmetrel) can produce
   a. constipation.
   b. mottling and swelling of the extremities.
   c. dyskinesias.
   d. sluggish pupillary response.

4. Which of the following is an adverse effect from levodopa that commonly occurs in the first few weeks of therapy?
   a. Hallucinations.
   b. Diarrhea.
   c. Hypotension.
   d. Urinary retention.

5. The physician plans to start your client on trihexyphenidyl (Artane). Which of the following assessments would warrant holding the medication until the physician had been contacted?
   a. Pulse of 102.
   b. BP of 88/60.
   c. Temperature of 100.2°.
   d. Respirations 14.

6. You should assess Mrs. C., who is receiving Sinemet (levodopa–carbidopa), for the following adverse reactions:
   a. Paralytic ileus.
   b. Gastrointestinal bleeding.
   c. Cardiac dysrhythmias.
   d. Hypotension.

7. Mr. P., age 75, is taking anticholinergic agents for Parkinson's disease and as a result is experiencing decreased sweating. This places him at a risk for experiencing
   a. dehydration.
   b. fluid volume overload.
   c. dry skin.
   d. heat stroke.

8. Which one of the following medications, if administered with levodopa–carbidopa (Sinemet), could increase its effects?
   a. Amantadine (Symmetrel).
   b. Diazepam (Valium).
   c. Reserpine (Serpasil).
   d. Alcohol.

9. Before administering benztropine (Cogentin), you should ask your client if he has a history of
   a. diabetes mellitus.
   b. glaucoma.
   c. peripheral vascular disease.
   d. pulmonary disease.

10. Anticholinergic drugs produce atropine-like effects such as
    a. tachycardia, constipation, and urinary retention.
    b. bradycardia, diarrhea, and diuresis.
    c. hypotension, lethargy, and angina.
    d. hypertension, constricted pupils, and ataxia.

CRITICAL THINKING CASE STUDY

Mr. P. is diagnosed with Parkinson's disease and started on benztropine (Cogentin), an anticholinergic agent.

1. Identify why Mr. P. was started on Cogentin.

2. Identify the adverse effects of this medication and the nursing measures that you will employ to prevent complications.

Three years after initial diagnosis, the medication Mr. P. is receiving is no longer effective and the physician starts Mr. P. on levodopa–carbidopa (Sinemet).

4. Discuss why this medication was chosen for Mr. P.

Mr. P. asks you about the progression of Parkinson's disease.

3. Describe how you will respond to his inquiry.

5. Identify what you will assess for and what you will teach the client.

13

Skeletal Muscle Relaxants

FILL IN THE BLANKS

Complete the following sentences.

1. Skeletal muscle relaxants are used to

   _____ or _____.

2. _____ is the only muscle relaxant that acts on the muscle itself.

3. Dantrolene (Dantrium) is also indicated for prevention and treatment of _____.

4. While taking muscle relaxants, clients should be
   instructed not to attempt activities that require

   _____ or _____.

5. The drug of choice for persons with multiple
   sclerosis is _____.

6. Which muscle relaxants can be given IV for
   acute muscle spasm? _____
   (_____), _____
   (_____), and _____
   (_____).

7. Adjunctive measures for muscle spasm include

   a. _____

   b. _____

   c. _____

   d. _____

   e. Regular exercise.

8. Muscle relaxants have not been established for

   safe use in _____.

9. Diazepam (Valium) should be administered at a
   rate of _____. This minimizes
   the risk of _____.

10. If methocarbamol (_____) is
    administered rapidly, it can cause

    _____, _____,

    and _____.

TRUE OR FALSE

1. _____ Dantrolene (Dantrium) is used for the
   treatment of malignant hyperthermia.

2. _____ If hypersensitivity reactions occur, the
   dosage of the drug should be decreased.

3. _____ Persons taking MAO inhibitors will need
   to increase their dose of muscle relaxants
   to produce the same effect.

4. _____ Diazepam (Valium) can produce psychological or physical dependence.

5. _____ The dosage of muscle relaxants should be
   increased slowly.

CROSSWORD PUZZLE

Across

2. An adverse effect of skeletal muscle relaxants.

3. Approved for treating people with multiple sclerosis.

4. A muscle relaxant that should be administered with food to prevent GI distress.

6. Persons with a spinal cord injury can experience _____.

8. The drug for prevention and treatment of malignant hyperthermia.

9. Skeletal muscle relaxants have not been proven safe for use during _____.

10. The patient should lie down while this drug is being administered via IV.

Down

1. A nonpharmacological intervention for muscle spasm.

5. Be cautious using this drug in persons with glaucoma or dysrhythmias.

7. Physically incompatible with other drugs of this class.

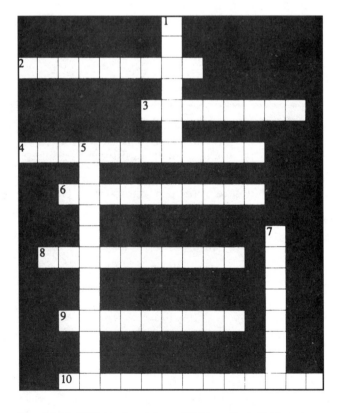

REVIEW QUESTIONS

1. Which of the following muscle relaxants is also used to treat malignant hyperthermia?

   a. Dantrolene (Dantrium).

   b. Diazepam (Valium).

   c. Baclofen (Lioresal).

   d. Carisoprodol (Soma).

2. The muscle relaxant of choice for persons who are pregnant is

   a. methocarbamol (Robaxin).

   b. diazepam (Valium).

   c. baclofen (Lioresal).

   d. none of the above.

3. A muscle relaxant that can be administered parenterally for acute muscle spasm is

   a. metaxalone (Skelaxin).

   b. baclofen (Lioresal).

   c. cyclobenzaprine (Flexeril).

   d. methocarbamol (Robaxin).

4. Which of the following statements indicates that your client, who is receiving dantrolene (Dantrium), has understood the teaching that you have done?

   a. "I will not stop my medication if I experience side effects. I will contact my physician."

   b. "I will limit my alcohol and caffeine intake while I am taking this medication."

   c. "The medicine may cause decreased tolerance to cold."

   d. "The medicine will prevent the progression of my multiple sclerosis."

5. Mr. H. is started on dantrolene (Dantrium) for muscle spasticity. Which of the following lab studies should be monitored when the medication is administered?

   a. Hematocrit and hemoglobin.

   b. SGOT and LDH.

   c. CPK (MB).

   d. Creatinine clearance.

6. The maximum recommended length of treatment with cyclobenzaprine (Flexeril) is

   a. 48–72 hours.

   b. 1 week.

   c. 2 weeks.

   d. 3 weeks.

7. Which of the following medications, if administered concurrently with muscle relaxants, will increase the risk of respiratory depression?

    a. Antihistamines.

    b. Antihypertensives.

    c. Antidiabetic agents.

    d. Diuretics.

8. When teaching Mrs. S. about the effects of baclofen (Lioresal), you should include the following information:

    a. The medication should be taken with milk or meals.

    b. You should expect a drop in your pulse rate.

    c. If you experience drowsiness, contact your physician immediately.

    d. Skin rashes are expected and will go away in a few weeks.

9. Cyclobenzaprine (Flexeril) should be used with caution for persons with the following conditions:

    a. Diabetes.

    b. Hypertension.

    c. Arthritis.

    d. Glaucoma.

10. Which of the following is an expected outcome when methocarbamol (Robaxin) is administered for acute muscle spasms?

    a. Increased tolerance to heat and cold.

    b. Increased physical coordination.

    c. Increased ability to maintain posture and balance.

    d. Increased mobility and decreased pain.

CRITICAL THINKING CASE STUDY

Joe Smith, a high school senior, injured his ankle in a football game. His physician ordered cyclobenzaprine (Flexeril) to relieve the pain associated with an ankle injury. Three weeks after his initial injury, he returned to his physician's office still complaining of pain and requesting a prescription renewal.

1. Identify the assessment that you will do.

2. Describe your response to his request for additional medication.

3. Discuss alternatives to drug therapy.

14

Anesthetics

MATCHING EXERCISE

Terms and Concepts

Match the concept with the term for it.

1. _____ One of the most widely used anesthetics.

2. _____ No longer used in the United States, still used in underdeveloped countries.

3. _____ Given intravenously to induce anesthesia.

4. _____ Given IM preoperatively for sedation.

5. _____ Its effects can be reversed by neostigmine.

6. _____ Its short duration of action makes it useful for endoscopy.

7. _____ Used in conjunction with general anesthesia (intermediate acting).

8. _____ Used alone for analgesia in dentistry, obstetrics, and brief surgical procedures.

9. _____ A very potent narcotic analgesic similar to morphine whose analgesic effect lasts about 30 minutes.

10. _____ A naturally occurring plant alkaloid that causes skeletal muscle paralysis.

11. _____ Given to prevent excessive activity of the parasympathetic nervous system.

12. _____ Administration of this drug preoperatively allows easier induction of anesthesia.

13. _____ Injection of an anesthetic solution around the area to be anesthetized.

14. _____ A solution used in spinal anesthesia that gravitates toward the head when the person is tilted in a head-down position.

15. _____ Topical anesthetic that has a rapid onset.

A. Ether.

B. Halothane (Fluothane).

C. Midazolam (Versed).

D. Fentanyl citrate (Sublimaze).

E. Thiopental sodium (Pentothal).

F. Tubocurarine.

G. Nitrous oxide.

H. Vercuronium (Norcuron).

I. Pancuronium (Pavulon).

J. Cyclopropane.

K. Succinylcholine (Anectine).

L. Glycopyrrolate (Robinul).

M. Hydroxyzine (Vistaril).

N. Field block.

O. Epidural anesthesia.

P. Vercuronium (Norevron).

Q. Hypobaric solution.

R. Lidocaine (Xylocaine).

WORD SCRAMBLE

Unscramble the word and circle it in the word find.

1. ranthee _____

2. nafoer _____

3. neatfal _____

4. ravionn _____

5. vonpaul _____

6. niceante _____

7. neetbium _____

8. falsentu _____

9. served _____

10. verbilat _____

Word Find

```
B A E C C T R I S O M E T A L C H E M P N I P A N
A L T B A C I T R E M E N A R C H O R O L A C O L
C M H T R A L C O H V P E R A G A R I R I H O K C
F O R A N E R L L S S N E S S T I T H E O P H Y L
T S A N S E I O E A A A N I N N O V A R E A N I X
O C N E T I P N E L A T I E N T G E O M T R I C U
B A E A L N P A L P I T F T I O N S E C O E S N E
A N E B O N D I H E X L L G H A L A B F I N I A X
C N U C T E C H Y P A V U L O N V E R E F L E X E
K A P T A B R A P P R E M E N E I O N T A O V A N
H A H S O M T R E M O R A N G C N E J T A O C N I
A B O T P E P I R N N Q B B A T T R I P C O C T N
N C R V Q T I H T E A B I E F I A R E S T L Y H H
E N I M O R B O E H T C N X O N T S E N I M A I C
C I A N S A N T N T A I N T M E T U B I N E M N Y
T A Y N A Z I T S L A E M O R D N F S S E T T E R
O M A H V O T R A C O M M R E X N E O E I F I N T
P P T A M L R T O P A M I N E C T N L B G N O I S
A H A A D O I C N A A F N N F D D T O E V E S O I
N A T I N V E R S E D I F A E L A A M M P A L O C
T I R E E E S T L E S S N E S S U A A W I T O O M
R R F R C S E T R E O N P I I A U N U T W R I M C
Y B B L R S H N V R R S I S E N I K R E P Y H C A
X T E L B E J Q U T H Y P O A C E B R S H I S P W
A L B E L L A D O W D Y M N T E S O O T Y P A K T
```

REVIEW QUESTIONS

1. Mr. J. was agitated and "fighting" the ventilator, so his physician ordered tubocurarine to help maintain Mr. J. on the ventilator. Now his physician wants the effects of the drug reversed. Which medication will be effective?

   a. Tetracaine (Pontocaine).

   b. Neostigmine.

   c. Thiopental sodium (Pentothal).

   d. Isoflurane (Forane).

2. Which of the following is a complication after general anesthesia that the nurse should be assessing for?

   a. Hypertension.

   b. Bradycardia.

   c. Urinary retention.

   d. Hypoxia.

3. An adverse effect of isoflurane (Forane) that the nurse needs to assess for is

   a. immobility.

   b. headache.

   c. blurred vision.

   d. depressed mental alertness.

4. After the use of a local anesthetic for mothers, a common side effect in babies immediately after delivery is

   a. depressed muscle tone.

   b. cyanosis.

   c. absent bowel sounds.

   d. inability to suck.

5. Before surgery, the anesthesiologist should be made aware of any medications that will decrease the effect of the general anesthetic agents. These medications include

   a. anticholinergic medications.

   b. bronchodilators.

   c. diuretics.

   d. antihypertensive medications.

6. The anesthesiologist plans on using methoxyflurane (Penthrane) for a C-section delivery. Because of the potential toxicity from this medication, you will assess which of the following lab values?

   a. Chloride.

   b. Blood sugar.

   c. Creatinine.

   d. Sodium.

7. Nitrous oxide is an anesthetic that has which of the following properties?

   a. Long recovery period.

   b. Many side effects.

   c. Short induction period.

   d. Explosive gas.

8. Stage II of general anesthesia is characterized by

   a. analgesia.

   b. medullary paralysis.

   c. surgical anesthesia.

   d. excitement and hyperactivity.

9. Before administering glycopyrrolate (Robinul) preoperatively, the nurse should ask the client if he or she has a history of the following condition:

   a. Glaucoma.

   b. Bradycardia.

   c. Hypertension.

   d. Diabetes mellitus.

10. As a result of the administration of general anesthetics, postoperative patients

    a. may have difficulty voiding and will have decreased gastric motility.

    b. need to be catheterized if they have not voided within 4 hours after surgery.

    c. need large amounts of oral fluids to flush the medication out of their system.

    d. should remain on bed rest to relieve abdominal pain and distention.

CRITICAL THINKING CASE STUDY

Mrs. J., a 29-year-old, is admitted for a C-section. Spinal anesthesia is performed.

1. Identify two other situations in which this type of anesthesia is the preferred method.

2. Mrs. J. asks you how long it will be after the surgery that she will be able to walk to the bathroom.

3. Mrs. J. asks you what she will be able to feel during surgery. Your response:

4. Specify fetal responses to anesthetics that the nurse should be assessing for.

5. Discuss nursing actions that are required in the event of an adverse response.

Mrs. J. has not voided 8 hours after delivery and is complaining of a headache.

6. Identify your nursing actions.

15

Alcohol and Other Drug Abuse

MATCHING EXERCISE

Terms and Concepts

Match the concept with the term for it.

1. _____ The primary drug of abuse worldwide.

2. _____ Symptoms of alcohol withdrawal.

3. _____ Symptoms of amphetamine withdrawal.

4. _____ Symptoms of barbiturate withdrawal.

5. _____ The use of this drug results in euphoric excitement and strong psychic dependence.

6. _____ A major danger with these drugs is their ability to impair judgement.

7. _____ These substances are most often abused by preadolescents.

8. _____ A potent analgesic that produces rapid, intense euphoria.

9. _____ This drug is used as an antiemetic for clients receiving anticancer drugs.

10. _____ A drug used in the treatment of alcohol abuse.

11. _____ A drug used in the treatment of heroin addiction.

12. _____ Symptoms seen with an overdose of opiate.

13. _____ Drug administered to reverse effects of an opiate.

14. _____ Drugs of choice for treating alcohol withdrawal.

15. _____ Treatment of an overdose of amphetamines includes these actions.

A. Cocaine.

B. Alcohol.

C. Tremors, sweating, nausea, tachycardia.

D. Heroin.

E. Depression and fatigue.

F. Hallucinogenic drugs.

G. Anxiety, tremors, insomnia, weight loss.

H. Marijuana.

I. Volatile solvent (inhalants).

J. Disulfiram (Antabuse).

K. Methadone (Dolophine).

L. Naloxone (Narcan).

M. Severe respiratory depression and coma.

N. Sedation, lowering of body temperature, administration of antipsychotic drugs.

O. Benzodiazepines.

NURSING DIAGNOSIS

Mr. Q., aged 29, is admitted with hepatic coma. Identify four nursing diagnoses, assessment data, and nursing interventions for a person requiring drug treatment for alcoholism.

1. Nursing Diagnosis:

   Assessment Data:

   Nursing Interventions:

2. Nursing Diagnosis:

   Assessment Data:

   Nursing Interventions:

3. Nursing Diagnosis:

   Assessment Data:

   Nursing Interventions:

4. Nursing Diagnosis:

   Assessment Data:

   Nursing Interventions:

DEFINITIONS

Define the following terms.

1. Alcoholism _____

   _____

2. Psychological dependence _____

   _____

3. Physical dependence _____

   _____

REVIEW QUESTIONS

1. Your client is started on disulfiram (Antabuse). You know that he has a good understanding of the side effects of the medication if he states

   a. "Antabuse can cause bruising. I'll contact my doctor if that happens."

   b. "It doesn't matter how much alcohol I drink, the reaction will be the same."

   c. "If I ingest alcohol with Antabuse, it can cause tachycardia, nausea, vomiting, and confusion."

   d. "I must always take Antabuse with meals to prevent nausea and vomiting."

2. Mr. J. is admitted to the emergency room with a cocaine overdose. The nurse should assess Mr. J. for

   a. dysrhythmia.

   b. congestion.

   c. hypotension.

   d. drowsiness.

3. Which of the following medications would be most effective in treating an overdose of morphine?

   a. Dronabinol (Marinol).

   b. Chloramphenicol (Chloromycetin).

   c. Disulfiram (Antabuse).

   d. Naloxone (Narcan).

4. Which of the following statements by Mr. C., a chronic alcoholic started on reserpine (Serpasil), leads you to believe that he has understood the teaching you have done regarding the medication?

   a. "If I drink alcohol with this medication, it may cause my blood pressure to go up."

   b. "If I drink alcohol, I must increase the amount of medication I am taking."

   c. "If I drink alcohol with this medication, it may cause my blood pressure to go down."

   d. "If I drink alcohol, I must decrease the amount of medication I am taking."

5. This drug is used as an antiemetic for persons receiving anticancer drugs.

   a. Cocaine.

   b. Marijuana.

   c. Heroin.

   d. PCP.

6. While Mr. G. is withdrawing from alcohol, you will

   a. encourage oral fluids to maintain hydration.

   b. withhold all medications.

   c. provide a nonstimulating environment.

   d. engage him in conversation to decrease his anxiety.

7. Mr. J. is admitted to the hospital following a car accident. He denies alcohol use, but the lab slip shows an alcohol level above the legal limit. The best approach to take is to

   a. wait until Mr. J. is ready to discuss his drinking problem.

   b. discuss the lab findings with Mr. J. and his family.

   c. confront Mr. J. with his alcohol abuse and persuade him to change.

   d. have a counselor come and see Mr. J.

8. Your client is admitted with acute amphetamine intoxication. You will observe her for

   a. somnolence and lethargy.

   b. bradycardia.

   c. hypothermia.

   d. hyperactivity and agitation.

9. A drug for treating alcohol withdrawal syndrome is

   a. naloxone (Narcan).

   b. methadone (Dolophine).

   c. disulfiram (Antabuse).

   d. clonazepam (Klonopin).

10. J.B. is admitted with intoxication from an unknown substance. He is hyperactive, tachycardic, febrile, and hallucinating. The symptoms probably relate to an overdose of

    a. amphetamines.

    b. barbiturates.

    c. alcohol.

    d. opiates.

CRITICAL THINKING CASE STUDY

M., a 28-year-old female, is admitted to your unit with symptoms of alcohol withdrawal. She was found on a park bench by the police. As a result of the admission blood work, you discover that M. is pregnant. (The learner may need additional resources to answer these questions.)

1. Describe how you will proceed with the admission history and physical of M.

2. Discuss how M.'s alcohol intake affects her pregnancy.

M. is anxious, agitated, and tremulous. Her vital signs are BP 90/60, pulse 100, and temperature 99.8°.

3. Discuss how M. will be treated for alcohol withdrawal.

4. Identify the symptoms of delirium tremens that the nurse should be assessing for.

You have observed that M. is a heavy smoker. She has now completed her treatment and is ready to go home.

5. Identify the information that you will give her before discharge.

6. You are concerned about M. and her baby. Describe the referrals you will make.

After delivery, M. plans to start disulfiram (Antabuse).

7. Identify the information that you will provide her.

16

Central Nervous System Stimulants

FILL IN THE BLANKS

1. Two disorders treated with CNS stimulants are _____ and _____.

2. Narcolepsy is _____ by periodic "sleep attacks."

3. Hyperkinetic syndrome occurs in _____ and is characterized by _____, _____, _____, _____, and _____.

4. Amphetamines produce _____ and _____. They also increase _____ and _____, produce _____, and slow _____. These drugs also produce _____ and _____.

5. Analeptic drugs stimulate _____. A major drawback is the adverse effect of _____.

6. Xanthine drugs increase _____ and decrease _____.

7. Xanthines also exacerbate _____, _____, _____, and _____.

8. Methylphenidate (_____) is used for children with ADHD. It is usually administered b.i.d. Monday through Friday while children are in school. The last dose each day should be given _____ hours before bedtime.

9. Doxapram (_____) increases tidal volume and respiratory rate. Duration of action of a single dose is _____ minutes.

10. Caffeine may increase _____. It may be combined with ergot alkaloids to treat _____.

11. Caffeine and sodium benzoate is used as a respiratory stimulant in _____.

12. Caffeine can produce _____, _____, or _____.

13. Children being treated for ADHD should avoid _____ in their diet.

14. Children receiving drugs for ADHD have reported suppression of _____ and _____.

15. Adverse effects of CNS stimulants include _____ _____ and _____ effects.

REVIEW QUESTIONS

1. A client, who is being treated for narcolepsy, must be assessed for adverse effects of dextroamphetamine (Dexedrine), which include
   a. impaired motor coordination.
   b. difficulty concentrating.
   c. muscle atrophy.
   d. altered growth and development.

2. An expected outcome when theophylline is administered is

   a. increased respiratory rate.

   b. increased tidal volume.

   c. bronchodilation.

   d. decreased oxygen demand.

3. When clients are receiving amphetamines, they should be assessed for

   a. weight loss.

   b. decreased urinary output.

   c. decreased pulse rate.

   d. bronchodilation.

4. The expected outcome when doxapram (Dopram) is administered is increased

   a. mental alertness.

   b. respiratory rate.

   c. cardiac output.

   d. oxygen use.

5. An amphetamine overdose can result in

   a. permanent memory loss.

   b. renal failure.

   c. convulsions.

   d. hepatic failure.

6. Which of the following statements by Mr. H. leads you to believe that he has understood the teaching you have done about methylphenidate (Ritalin)?

   a. "Over the counter medication has no impact on this medication."

   b. "It produces tolerance, and habituation can occur."

   c. "There are no adverse effects with this medication."

   d. "It should not be taken within 6–8 hours of bedtime."

7. When caffeine is administered with the following drug, it will increase its effect:

   a. Theophylline.

   b. Cimetidine (Tagamet).

   c. Propranolol (Inderal).

   d. Furosemide (Lasix).

8. Caffeine is found in all of these over the counter medications *except*

   a. Excedrin.

   b. Vanquish.

   c. No-Doz.

   d. Tylenol.

9. This drug is used as a respiratory stimulant in neonates who are experiencing apnea that is unresponsive to other treatments.

   a. Dextroamphetamine (Dexedrine).

   b. Doxapram (Dopram).

   c. Caffeine and sodium benzoate.

   d. Methamphetamine (Desoxyn).

10. The use of central nervous system stimulants is contraindicated in persons with the following disorders:

    a. Depression.

    b. Hyperthyroidism.

    c. Chronic obstructive pulmonary disease.

    d. Diabetes mellitus.

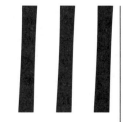

DRUGS AFFECTING THE AUTONOMIC NERVOUS SYSTEM

17

Physiology of the Autonomic Nervous System

FILL IN THE BLANKS

Use the following terms to fill in the blanks in the Autonomic Nervous System table. Each term may be used more than once.

Increases   Decreases   Constricts   Dilates   Contracts   Relaxes

Autonomic Nervous System

PARASYMPATHETIC RESPONSE	BODY TISSUE/ ORGAN	SYMPATHETIC RESPONSE		
		Alpha₁	Beta₁	Beta₂
1. _____	Blood vessels	8. _____		
2. _____ rate	Heart		10. _____ rate	
3. _____ contraction			11. _____ contraction	
4. _____	Lungs			12. _____
5. _____ motility	GI			13. _____ motility
6. _____	Eye	9. _____		
7. _____	Bladder			14. _____

TRUE OR FALSE

1. _____ Anticholinergic drugs act by blocking the action of acetylcholine.

2. _____ Cholinergic drugs produce bronchoconstriction.

3. _____ Adrenergic drugs decrease myocardial contractility.

4. _____ Adrenergic drugs may be used in the treatment of tachycardia.

5. _____ Beta-adrenergic blocking agents are given for bronchodilating effects.

6. _____ Beta-blocking drugs may cause tachycardia.

REVIEW QUESTIONS

1. When nonselective beta-adrenergic blocking drugs are administered, they increase the person's risk of
   a. hypertension.
   b. acute myocardial infarction.
   c. asthma.
   d. atrial fibrillation.

2. An expected outcome with the administration of beta-adrenergic blocking agents is
   a. increased cardiac output.
   b. increased oxygen consumption.
   c. increased blood pressure.
   d. decreased exercise tolerance.

3. Drugs that stimulate the parasympathetic nervous system cause
   a. decreased sweating.
   b. increased heart rate.
   c. pupillary constriction.
   d. dilation of bronchi.

4. Alpha-adrenergic blocking agents may affect
   a. platelet aggregation.
   b. lipolysis.
   c. release of renin.
   d. glycogenolysis.

5. An agent developed to stimulate beta$_2$ receptors to produce bronchodilation without tachycardia.
   a. Isoproterenol (Isuprel).
   b. Isoetharine (Bronkosol).
   c. Xylometazoline hydrochloride (Otrivin).
   d. Terbutaline (Brethine).

6. When an adrenergic agent is administered it will
   a. decrease arterial blood pressure.
   b. increase blood sugar.
   c. decrease muscle strength.
   d. increase gastric motility.

7. When anticholinergic agents are administered the nurse should assess the client for
   a. tachycardia.
   b. diarrhea.
   c. clotting disorders.
   d. hypoglycemia.

8. An expected outcome of the administration of cholinergic drugs is
   a. increased muscle strength.
   b. increased blood pressure.
   c. increased gastric motility.
   d. increased heart rate.

9. A beta-adrenergic blocker should be administered with caution to persons who have this disorder.
   a. Hypertension.
   b. Angina.
   c. Heart failure.
   d. Atrial flutter.

10. Which of the following agents inhibit parasympathetic stimulation?
    a. Adrenergic agents.
    b. Antiadrenergic agents.
    c. Cholinergic agents.
    d. Anticholinergic agents.

18

Adrenergic Drugs

A. Isoproterenol (Isuprel).

B. Narrow-angle glaucoma.

C. Dopamine (Intropin).

D. Dobutamine (Dobutrex).

E. Epinephrine (Adrenalin).

F. Albuterol (Proventil).

G. Caffeine.

H. Phenylpropanolamine hydrochloride (Propagest).

I. Pseudoephedrine (Sudafed).

J. Bronkaid Mist.

MATCHING EXERCISE

Terms and Concepts

Match the concept with the term for it.

1. _____ A drug used to raise the blood pressure.

2. _____ An intravenous medication used to increase the force of the contraction of the heart.

3. _____ This drug produces bronchodilation and increases the heart rate.

4. _____ Commonly used inhaler that produces bronchodilation.

5. _____ This drug is used for the treatment of allergic reactions, shock, and cardiac arrest.

6. _____ A contraindication for the use of adrenergic agents.

7. _____ This drug is used for bronchodilation and nasal congestion and is sold over the counter.

8. _____ This substance has a synergistic bronchodilating effect when administered with adrenergic agents.

9. _____ This drug, used for nasal congestion, also acts as an appetite suppressant.

10. _____ Can lose its effectiveness with prolonged use.

TRUE OR FALSE

1. _____ Epinephrine (Adrenalin) causes peripheral vasoconstriction and bronchodilation.

2. _____ Common adverse effects from the administration of adrenergic drugs include hypotension and bradycardia.

3. _____ Albuterol (Proventil) should not be given to children under 12 years of age.

4. _____ An expected outcome of the administration of dopamine (Intropin) is increased urinary output.

5. _____ Inhaled solutions of isoproterenol (Isuprel) may turn saliva pink.

6. _____ When nasal decongestants are used excessively, a rebound nasal congestion can result.

7. _____ When adrenergic agents are administered with beta-blockers, the effect of the adrenergic agent is increased.

8. _____ Epinephrine (Adrenalin) can only be administered parenterally.

9. _____ A common side effect from the administration of epinephrine (Adrenalin) is elevated serum glucose.

10. _____ The usual goal of vasopressor therapy is to maintain the systolic blood pressure above 80.

SENTENCE CORRECTION

Circle the word that makes the sentence incorrect and place the correct word in the space provided. Example:
increases Dobutamine (Dobutrex) (decreases) cardiac output.

1. _____ Ephedrine is used as a bronchodilator to treat bronchospasm.

2. _____ An allergic reaction produces severe respiratory distress and profound hypertension.

3. _____ Acute asthma attacks may be precipitated by exposure to toxins.

4. _____ Alkalosis may occur with acute bronchospasm.

5. _____ When administering substances known to produce hypersensitivity reactions, observe the recipient carefully for 5 minutes after administration.

6. _____ Levarterenol (Levophed) stimulates electrical and mechanical activity to produce myocardial contraction.

7. _____ Ephedrine is used to treat Marfan syndrome, a sudden attack of unconsciousness brought on by heart block.

8. _____ Pseudoephedrine is an ingredient in cold medications.

9. _____ Isoproterenol (Isuprel) may cause chest pain and bradycardia.

10. _____ Terbutaline (Brethine) is not recommended for children over the age of 12.

11. _____ When giving dopamine (Intropin) observe for improved breathing.

12. _____ The use of excessive amounts of nasal decongestants can result in hypertension.

13. _____ When assessing for the effectiveness of vasopressors, you should assess blood pressures and the person's respiratory status.

14. _____ Anticholinergic drugs decrease the effects of adrenergic drugs.

15. _____ Metaraminol (Aramine) is used for bronchodilation and vasoconstriction in the eye.

REVIEW QUESTIONS

1. The use of adrenergic drugs is contraindicated in persons with the following condition:
   a. Diabetes mellitus.
   b. Tachycardia.
   c. Hypotension.
   d. Bronchoconstriction.

2. An expected outcome after the administration of dopamine (Intropin) is
   a. increased blood pressure.
   b. headache.
   c. decreased pulse.
   d. decreased respirations.

3. The drug of choice for treating spinal shock is
   a. ephedrine.
   b. dopamine (Intropin).
   c. dobutamine (Dobutrex).
   d. epinephrine (Adrenalin).

4. Your client has a cardiac arrest and is given epinephrine (Adrenalin). After his condition is stabilized, blood work is drawn and the results are glucose 160, WBC 5000, PTT 15 seconds, K 5.0 mEq/liter. Which deviation in these lab values is attributable to the use of epinephrine (Adrenalin)?
   a. WBC.
   b. Glucose.
   c. PTT.
   d. Potassium.

5. Which of the following comments by Mr. J.'s wife leads you to believe that she has a good understanding of why her husband is receiving terbutaline (Brethine): "The doctor ordered the medication to. . . ."
   a. "increase the force of the contraction of my husband's heart."
   b. "decrease my husband's pCO_2."
   c. "improve his oxygen exchange."
   d. "decrease his oxygen requirements."

6. After a breathing treatment with isoproterenol (Isuprel) your client calls you into her room stating, "My heart is racing; I think something is wrong." Your best response would be

   a. "Lie down and rest and I will take your vital signs in 15 minutes."

   b. "I will contact your physician immediately."

   c. "An increased pulse rate is common when isoproterenol (Isuprel) is given by inhalation."

   d. "You have no need to be alarmed. This is a common side effect."

7. Which of the following medications, if administered concurrently with adrenergic drugs, will decrease their effect?

   a. Beta-adrenergic blockers.

   b. Xanthines.

   c. Anticholinergics.

   d. Tricyclic antidepressants.

8. Your client with COPD who is taking albuterol (Proventil) needs to be observed for

   a. anxiety, nervousness, and insomnia.

   b. bradycardia and hypotension.

   c. fluid retention.

   d. bronchoconstriction.

9. Ephedrine works by

   a. stimulating the release of norepinephrine.

   b. blocking beta receptors.

   c. blocking alpha receptors.

   d. stimulating the release of acetylcholine.

10. When using a vasopressor, the goal of therapy is to maintain the systolic blood pressure at

    a. 40–50 mmHg.

    b. 60–70 mmHg.

    c. 80–100 mmHg.

    d. 120–140 mmHg.

CRITICAL THINKING CASE STUDY

Mr. J. had a myocardial infarction this morning. The physician orders IV drips of dopamine (Intropin) and lidocaine (Xylocaine). (The learner may need to use additional sources to answer these questions.)

1. Explain why these drugs were ordered.

2. Identify what nursing assessments you will be performing and your rationale for each.

Mr. J. develops right-sided heart failure. The physician adds dobutamine (Dobutrex) to the medical regime.

3. Explain why this drug was added to the medical regime and the expected therapeutic effect.

Mr. J.'s condition deteriorates. His heart rate drops to 40 and the physician orders isoproterenol (Isuprel).

4. Identify why this medication was chosen by the physician and the side effects of the medication that you will be assessing for.

5. If these medications do not effectively treat Mr. J.'s heart failure, what other measures could be instituted?

19

Antiadrenergic Drugs

A. Labetalol (Trandate).

B. Atenolol (Tenormin).

C. Difficulty in breathing.

D. Propranolol (Inderal).

E. Esmolol (Brevibloc).

F. Betaxolol (Betoptic).

G. Digoxin (Lanoxin).

H. Prazosin (Minipress).

I. Acebutolol (Sectral).

J. Isoproterenol (Isuprel).

K. Blurred vision.

MATCHING EXERCISE

Terms and Concepts

Match the concept with the term for it.

1. _____ Used for the treatment of supraventricular tachycardia.

2. _____ This drug is valuable in the treatment of glaucoma.

3. _____ The drug of choice for treating hypertensive emergencies.

4. _____ Clients use this drug to prevent migraine headaches.

5. _____ A selective beta-blocker used to treat a myocardial infarction.

6. _____ This can result when nonselective beta-blockers are administered.

7. _____ This drug is effective in treating ventricular arrhythmias.

8. _____ When this drug is administered with beta-adrenergic blockers, heart block can result.

9. _____ An alpha-adrenergic antagonist used for the treatment of hypertension.

10. _____ When this drug is administered concurrently with beta-adrenergic blockers, it will decrease the effect of the beta-adrenergic blocking agent.

TRUE OR FALSE

1. _____ Beta-adrenergic blockers increase oxygen consumption.

2. _____ Beta-blockers act to prevent sympathetic nervous system stimulation of various organs and tissues.

3. _____ Beta-blockers decrease the force of myocardial contraction, decrease cardiac output, decrease blood pressure, and decrease heart rate.

4. _____ Beta-blockers are apparently equally effective in the treatment of hypertension.

5. _____ Major adverse effects of beta-blockers are congestive heart failure, bradycardia, and bronchospasm.

6. _____ Adverse effects of beta-adrenergic blockers include CNS problems (e.g., nervousness, insomnia, hallucinations, mental depression) and sexual dysfunction (impotence, decreased libido).

7. _____ Metoprolol (Lopressor), atenolol (Tenormin), and acebutolol (Sectral) are cardioselective.

8. _____ Propranolol (Inderal) is used in the treatment of hypertension, angina pectoris, and cardiac dysrhythmias.

9. _____ Atenolol (Tenormin), metoprolol (Lopressor), propranolol (Inderal), and timolol (Blocadren) are approved for use in prevention of reinfarction.

10. _____ Two oral beta-adrenergic blockers should not be administered concurrently.

SENTENCE CORRECTION

Circle the word that makes the sentence incorrect and place the correct word in the space provided. Example: Esmolol (Brevibloc) Propranolol is used to treat supraventricular tachycardia.

1. _____ Nadolol (Corgard) is the oldest of the beta-blocking agents.

2. _____ Acebutolol (Sectral) is a nonselective beta-blocker used to treat hypertension.

3. _____ Esmolol (Brevibloc) is the drug of choice for treating hypertension.

4. _____ A nonselective beta-blocker used to treat glaucoma is pindolol (Visken).

5. _____ The beta-blocker of choice for treating migraine headaches is levobunolol (Betagan).

6. _____ Metoprolol (Lopressor) is an alpha-blocker used for the treatment of hypertensive emergencies.

7. _____ A cardioselective beta-blocker used for the treatment of angina is penbutolol (Levatol).

8. _____ Selective beta-blockers should not be used for persons with respiratory diseases.

9. _____ A nonselective beta-blocker used for the treatment of a myocardial infarction is levobunolol (Betagan).

10. _____ Beta-adrenergic blocking agents are contraindicated when the individual has had a stroke.

11. _____ Timolol (Timoptic) reduces intraocular pressure by increasing the formation of aqueous humor.

12. _____ The term "selective" indicates that those drugs have more effect on beta$_2$ receptors.

13. _____ Beta-blockers are likely to cause tachycardia.

14. _____ Beta-blockers that are highly water soluble are more likely to cause depression, nightmares, insomnia, and hallucinations.

15. _____ In the presence of hepatic disease, the dosage of timolol should be increased.

REVIEW QUESTIONS

1. Mr. P. has hypertension and a ventricular dysrhythmia. Which of the following beta-adrenergic blocking agents would be most effective for him.?
   a. Acebutolol (Sectral).
   b. Atenolol (Tenormin).
   c. Esmolol (Brevibloc).
   d. Metoprolol (Lopressor).

2. Which of the following beta-adrenergic blocking agents would be most effective in treating supraventricular tachycardia?
   a. Propranolol (Inderal).
   b. Nadolol (Corgard).
   c. Esmolol (Brevibloc).
   d. Acebutolol (Sectral).

3. Beta-adrenergic blocking agents will
   a. increase glucose production.
   b. decrease cardiac perfusion.
   c. increase cardiac output.
   d. decrease oxygen consumption.

4. Mr. C. is receiving propranolol (Inderal) for migraine headaches. It is important to assess Mr. C.'s pulse rate and to examine his lab studies for a possible drop in
   a. serum potassium.
   b. WBC.
   c. blood sugar.
   d. hemoglobin.

5. Which of the following statements by Mrs. H. leads you to believe that she understands the teaching that you have done regarding atenolol (Tenormin)?
   a. "If I experience side effects, I will stop taking the medication."
   b. "I am not allowed to have any caffeine."
   c. "Smoking will not reduce the effectiveness of the medication."
   d. "I will take my pulse daily."

6. The following drug, when administered with propranolol (Inderal), will decrease the effect of Inderal:
   a. Atropine.
   b. Digoxin (Lanoxin).
   c. Phenytoin (Dilantin).
   d. Quinidine.

7. Which of the following instructions should be included when you are discharging a client on metoprolol (Lopressor)?

   a. When taking this drug, you should exercise strenuously 30 minutes a day.

   b. Report weight loss of more than 2 lb in 1 week.

   c. Take the medication on an empty stomach to enhance its absorption.

   d. Ingestion of alcohol with this drug can cause dizziness.

8. In reviewing Mr. J.'s history, you discover that he has a history of diabetes mellitus, myocardial infarction, multiple sclerosis, and peptic ulcer disease. Which one of the diagnoses above would you discuss with the physician before administering a beta-adrenergic blocker?

   a. Myocardial infarction.

   b. Multiple sclerosis.

   c. Diabetes mellitus.

   d. Peptic ulcer disease.

9. When a nonselective beta-blocker is administered, there is a greater risk of

   a. bronchoconstriction.

   b. reflex tachycardia.

   c. respiratory depression.

   d. arrhythmias.

10. Which of the following medications, if administered with labetalol (Trandate), will increase its effect?

    a. Epinephrine.

    b. Levarterenol (Levophed).

    c. Atropine.

    d. Phenytoin (Dilantin).

CRITICAL THINKING CASE STUDY

Your client Mary is a 54-year-old female diagnosed with essential hypertension. Her blood pressure is 140/90. Her physician places her on propranolol (Inderal).

1. Identify the teaching that you will do with Mary that will help her control her hypertension.

2. Identify the concurrent medical diagnosis that would preclude the use of Inderal.

After 2 months Mary returns and her blood pressure is still elevated and her physician adds Hydrodiuril to her regime.

3. Identify the rationale for the multiple drug regime.

Discuss the adverse effects associated with each medication.

4. Identify the objective assessments that will be important when monitoring Mary.

20

Cholinergic Drugs

A. Used as an antidote for tubocurarine.

B. Used to diagnose myasthenia gravis.

C. Used to treat Alzheimer disease.

D. Used for urinary retention and paralytic ileus.

E. Used as an antidote for "atropine poisoning."

FILL IN THE BLANKS

Use the following terms to fill in the blanks. Each term may be used more than once.

increased   decreased

relaxation of   constriction of

1. Direct-acting cholinergic drugs cause

   a. _____ heart rate.

   b. _____ contractility of gastrointestinal smooth muscle.

   c. _____ sphincters.

   d. _____ contractility of smooth muscle of the bladder.

   e. _____ contractility of bronchial smooth muscle.

   f. _____ respiratory secretions.

   g. _____ pupils.

MATCHING EXERCISE

Terms and Concepts

Match the drug with its action.

1. ____ Bethanechol (Urecholine).

2. ____ Neostigmine (Prostigmin).

3. ____ Edrophonium (Tensilon).

4. ____ Tacrine (Cognex).

5. ____ Physostigmine salicylate (Antilirium).

TRUE OR FALSE

1. ____ The dosage of anticholinesterase drugs may need to be increased if the client develops an infection.

2. ____ Bethanechol (Urecholine) should be administered with meals.

3. ____ Hypertension is a common side effect of cholinergic drugs.

4. ____ When antihistamines are administered concurrently with cholinergic drugs, they decrease the effect of the cholinergic drug.

5. ____ Pyridostigmine (Mestinon) is taken at bedtime to prevent the client from experiencing an inability to swallow upon awakening.

REVIEW QUESTIONS

1. Your client asks you why his physician ordered bethanechol (Urecholine) for him postoperatively. The best response is to explain that Bethanechol (Urecholine) is administered postoperatively to

   a. improve gastric motility.

   b. decrease adventitious breath sounds.

   c. decrease abdominal discomfort.

   d. increase urinary output.

2. An expected outcome after administration of pyridostigmine for myasthenia gravis is

   a. improved appetite.

   b. fewer headaches.

   c. increased muscle strength.

   d. decreased tremors.

3. The physician has ordered neostigmine (Prostigmin) for a client with paraplegia to

   a. increase bladder capacity.

   b. increase urinary output.

   c. increase muscle strength.

   d. prevent constipation.

4. Which of the following anticholinergic drugs is the drug of choice for a tubocurarine overdose?

    a. Bethanechol (Urecholine).

    b. Neostigmine (Prostigmin).

    c. Edrophonium (Tensilon).

    d. Physostigmine salicylate (Antilirium).

5. Which of the following statements by your client leads you to believe that she has understood the teaching you have done regarding pyridostigmine (Mestinon)?

    a. "I will limit my fluid intake to 1500 cc while I am taking this medication."

    b. "If I have increased sweating, I will contact the doctor immediately."

    c. "It is important that I take this medication on time."

    d. "I will take the medication with meals."

6. The antidote the physician should have on hand when he or she is administering edrophonium (Tensilon) is

    a. atropine.

    b. dopamine (Intropin).

    c. phenytoin (Dilantin).

    d. epinephrine.

7. When you are administering bethanechol (Urecholine) to Mr. B., you should observe him for evidence of a cholinergic crisis. Symptoms include

    a. hypertension.

    b. confusion.

    c. fever.

    d. respiratory failure.

8. For which of the following disorders is the use of cholinergics contraindicated?

    a. Hypertension.

    b. Parkinson's disease.

    c. Diabetes mellitus.

    d. Peptic ulcer disease.

9. An adverse effect after administration of cholinergic agents is increased

    a. heart rate.

    b. serum glucose level.

    c. blood pressure.

    d. respiratory secretions.

10. Which of the following instructions should you give Mr. G., who is starting on bethanechol (Urecholine)?

    a. Avoid foods high in vitamin C.

    b. Increase your fluid intake to 3000 cc a day.

    c. Increase the roughage in your diet.

    d. Take the medication before meals.

CRITICAL THINKING CASE STUDY

J., a 9-year-old weighing 66 lb, is admitted to your unit following surgery for a ruptured appendix. He has an NG tube to suction intermittently and a Foley catheter in place. No bowel sounds are auscultated. (The learner may need to use additional sources to answer the questions below.)

1. Discuss why it is common for there to be no bowel sounds after abdominal surgery and when you can expect bowel sounds to return.

2. Identify the electrolyte imbalances you should be assessing for.

Three days after surgery, J.'s abdomen is distended and he has only faint hypoactive bowel sounds and he is having difficulty voiding. The physician orders bethanechol (Urecholine) 5 mg q.i.d.

3. Identify why the physician ordered this medication and whether the dose the physician ordered is within the therapeutic range for J.

You go into J.'s room to administer his morning dose of bethanechol (Urecholine) and find that his pupils are constricted. His pulse is 110, respirations 16, BP 80/60, and temperature 102°. J. complains of a headache and nausea. You notice that his bed is wet from perspiration.

5. Identify which signs/symptoms from your assessment are directly related to the cholinergic drug he is taking and what your nursing actions will be.

4. Identify the expected outcome after this medication is administered.

J. becomes short of breath.

6. Identify and prioritize your nursing actions.

21

Anticholinergic Drugs

FILL IN THE BLANKS

Complete the following sentences.

1. Anticholinergic drugs block the action of
   _____ on the _____
   nervous system.

2. The effects that anticholinergic drugs have on
   the body include
   a. _____
   b. _____
   c. _____
   d. _____
   e. _____
   f. _____
   g. _____
   h. _____

3. GI disorders for which anticholinergics are useful include _____,
   _____, _____,
   _____, _____,
   and _____.

4. Anticholinergics are used in ophthalmology to
   aid in _____ or
   _____ because they produce
   _____ and _____
   effects.

5. Atropine is given to _____ the
   heart rate.

6. When a client is experiencing bronchoconstriction, ipratropium (Atrovent) may be given by
   _____.

7. Anticholinergic drugs are used with clients who
   have enuresis, paraplegia, or neurogenic bladder
   to _____.

8. Atropine and glycopyrrolate (Robinul) are used
   preoperatively to reduce _____
   and to prevent _____.

9. Contraindications for the use of anticholinergic
   drugs include _____,
   _____, _____,
   _____, and _____
   unless bradycardia is present.

10. Atropine is the _____ PO anti-
    cholinergic drug and can be administered
    _____, _____,
    _____, _____,
    and by _____.

11. Hyoscyamine (Anaspaz) is a belladonna alkaloid
    used for gastrointestinal and urinary tract disor-
    ders that cause _____,
    _____, and _____.

12. Scopolamine is also used for
    _____. It can be administered
    orally and as a _____, and it is
    effective for _____ hours.

13. _____ (Artane) is used for ini-
    tial treatment of _____. It is
    also effective in treating _____
    caused by antipsychotic drugs.

14. _____ (Cogentin) is used for
    prevention and treatment of _____.

15. Flavoxate (Urispas) relieves _____,

    _____, _____,

    and _____.

16. Oxybutynin (_____) increases

    _____ and decreases

    _____.

17. Anticholinergic drugs are used to treat

    a. _____

    b. _____

    c. _____

    d. _____

    e. _____

    f. _____

    g. _____

18. The antidote for an atropine overdose is

    _____ (_____).

19. Adverse responses to anticholinergic agents seen

    in children include _____ and

    _____.

20. Common adverse reactions from anticholinergic

    drugs that the elderly experience include

    _____, _____,

    _____, _____,

    _____, _____,

    and _____.

TRUE OR FALSE

1. _____ Meperidine (Demerol) and atropine cannot be mixed in the same syringe.

2. _____ Saunas should be avoided by persons taking anticholinergic drugs.

3. _____ Anticholinergic drugs are used to produce pupillary constriction.

4. _____ Persons taking anticholinergics for peptic ulcer disease should also drink large amounts of milk to decrease gastric acid secretion.

5. _____ Dental caries and loss of teeth can occur from decreased saliva production due to administration of anticholinergic drugs.

MATCHING EXERCISE

Match the generic and trade names of the anticholinergic drugs.

1. _____ Urispas.

2. _____ Cogentin.

3. _____ Robinul.

4. _____ Anaspaz.

5. _____ Ditropan.

6. _____ Probanthine.

A. Glycopyrrolate.

B. Hyoscyamine.

C. Flavoxate.

D. Benztropine.

E. Oxybutynin.

F. Propantheline bromide.

REVIEW QUESTIONS

1. A client asks you why his physician ordered glycopyrrolate (Robinul) for him preoperatively. Your best response is to explain that glycopyrrolate (Robinul) is administered preoperatively to

   a. prevent hypertension.

   b. decrease adventitious breath sounds.

   c. decrease respiratory tract secretions.

   d. increase urinary output.

2. An expected outcome after administration of trihexyphenidyl (Artane) for Parkinson's disease is

   a. improved appetite.

   b. fewer headaches.

   c. a regular gait.

   d. decreased tremors.

3. Persons taking anticholinergic medications are susceptible to heat exhaustion and should do the following to minimize that risk:

    a. Eat a diet high in sodium.

    b. Exercise 30 minutes a day in the morning or evening.

    c. Take cool baths and wear cool clothing.

    d. Avoid going outside.

4. Mr. J. is started on trihexyphenidyl (Artane) for treatment of Parkinson's disease. Which of the following instructions should he be given?

    a. This medication should be taken once a day at bedtime.

    b. Take this medication on an empty stomach.

    c. You may experience mouth dryness from this medication.

    d. This medication will stop the progression of the disease.

5. Mrs. G. is having extrapyramidal symptoms caused by the phenothiazines she is taking. Which of the following anticholinergic agents would be most effective in treating her symptoms?

    a. Homatropine methylbromide (Homapin).

    b. Hyoscyamine (Anaspaz).

    c. Methscopolamine (Pamine).

    d. Trihexyphenidyl (Artane).

6. Oxybutynin (Ditropan) is being given to a client to increase his bladder capacity. A side effect of this medication that would be significant for someone with paraplegia is

    a. weight gain.

    b. lethargy.

    c. dizziness.

    d. constipation.

7. Which of the following medications would be most effective in treating an atropine overdose?

    a. Physostigmine salicylate (Antilirium).

    b. Dopamine (Intropin).

    c. Phenytoin (Dilantin).

    d. Epinephrine.

8. Inadvertently, your client was given two preoperative injections of Demerol 100 mg IM and atropine 0.25 mg IM. The following adverse reactions are most likely to occur as a result of an atropine overdose:

    a. Increased respiratory secretions.

    b. Heat stroke and vomiting.

    c. Urinary retention and decreased intestinal motility.

    d. Hypotension and bradycardia.

9. An expected outcome after administration of high doses of atropine is

    a. increased heart rate.

    b. elevated blood glucose level.

    c. decreased blood pressure.

    d. increased respiratory rate.

10. After receiving atropine, Mrs. J. complains of eye pain. You know that this may be indicative of

    a. a common harmless reaction to the medication.

    b. increased intraocular pressure.

    c. excessive CNS stimulation.

    d. CNS depression.

CRITICAL THINKING CASE STUDY

Mr. P., a 76-year-old man with heart failure, is brought to the hospital because he fainted at home. He has been taking digoxin (Lanoxin), furosemide (Lasix), and KCl (potassium chloride) for 5 years. He is alert and oriented but weak. When you check Mr. P.'s apical pulse, you find it to be 40. The physician diagnoses heart block and administers atropine. Soon after the administration of atropine, Mr. P. becomes agitated and confused. (The learner may need to use additional sources to answer the questions below.)

1. Identify and prioritize your nursing actions.

Mr. P. is complaining of a dry mouth and blurred vision.

2. Describe your response to Mr. P.

Mr. P.'s physician decides to insert a pacemaker. Mr. P. states "now I will no longer need to take medication for my heart failure."

3. Specify the best response.

IV

DRUGS AFFECTING THE ENDOCRINE SYSTEM

22

Physiology of the Endocrine System

A. Parathyroid hormone.

B. Glucagon.

C. Testicular hormone.

D. ADH.

E. Glucocorticoids.

F. Mineralocorticoid.

G. Estrogen.

H. Progesterone.

I. Epinephrine.

J. Thyroid hormones.

K. Cholecystokinin.

L. Erythropoietin.

MATCHING EXERCISE

Terms and Concepts

Match the concept with the term for it.

1. _____ Helps maintain fluid balance.

2. _____ Influence carbohydrate storage.

3. _____ Promotes sodium retention and potassium loss.

4. _____ The adrenal medulla secretes this hormone.

5. _____ These hormones regulate the metabolic rate of the body.

6. _____ This hormone regulates calcium and phosphate metabolism.

7. _____ Regulates the metabolism of glucose, lipids, and proteins.

8. _____ Promotes the development of secondary sex characteristics in females.

9. _____ Regulates the development of male characteristics.

10. _____ Helps prepare the mammary glands for lactation.

11. _____ Stimulates bone marrow to produce RBCs.

12. _____ A hormone that is important in digestion.

TRUE OR FALSE

1. _____ The length of the physiological effects of the endocrine hormone varies from minutes to hours.

2. _____ All hormones are secreted by the pituitary gland.

3. _____ Cancerous tumors can produce hormones.

4. _____ Steroid hormones are synthesized from amino acids.

5. _____ Secretion of all pituitary hormones is controlled by the hypothalamus.

REVIEW QUESTIONS

1. Along with insulin, the pancreatic hormone that helps regulate the metabolism of glucose is

   a. epinephrine.

   b. lactogen.

   c. cortisol.

   d. glucagon.

2. The secretion of pituitary hormone is controlled by the

   a. hypothalamus.

   b. anterior pituitary.

   c. posterior pituitary.

   d. thalamus.

3. The antidiuretic hormone is released in response to
   a. increased blood pressure.
   b. increased serum sodium levels.
   c. decreased plasma protein.
   d. increased blood pressure.

4. ADH is secreted by the
   a. anterior pituitary.
   b. posterior pituitary.
   c. thyroid gland.
   d. parathyroid gland.

5. Mineralocorticoids help regulate
   a. electrolyte balance.
   b. metabolism of glucose, lipids, and proteins.
   c. the development of feminine characteristics.
   d. carbohydrate storage and protein catabolism.

6. Adrenal medulla hormones that affect the heart rate and blood pressure are
   a. cortisol and aldosterone.
   b. gastrin and enterogastrone.
   c. secretin and cholecystokinin.
   d. epinephrine and norepinephrine.

7. An insulin-dependent diabetic is started on a glucocorticoid. The addition of this medication
   a. will have no effect on his insulin requirements.
   b. may increase his insulin requirements.
   c. may decrease his insulin requirements.
   d. is likely to cause a toxic effect that must be carefully assessed for.

8. Your client's parathyroid gland was inadvertently removed during surgery. You should assess him for
   a. respiratory distress.
   b. tetany.
   c. hypertension.
   d. sodium retention.

9. Erythropoietin
   a. stimulates the bone marrow to produce RBCs.
   b. stimulates the growth of bones and muscles.
   c. regulates the osmolality of extracellular fluids.
   d. promotes sodium and water retention.

10. A type II diabetic is reluctant to start on insulin. Your best response would be
   a. "Insulin helps regulate the metabolism of glucose, something that your body is no longer able to do."
   b. "Insulin helps regulate the growth of bone and muscle cells and will prevent you from getting fractures in the future."
   c. "Insulin raises blood glucose levels by promoting the breakdown of glycogen in the liver; without the medication this would not be possible."
   d. "Insulin regulates the osmolality of the extracellular fluid. Without insulin you would retain fluid."

23

Hypothalamic and Pituitary Hormones

MATCHING EXERCISE

Terms and Concepts

Match the concept with the term for it.

1. _____ The posterior pituitary.

2. _____ Stimulates functions of sex glands.

3. _____ Plays a role in skin pigmentation.

4. _____ Plays a part in milk production in nursing mothers.

5. _____ Causes reabsorption of water.

6. _____ Excessive production of this hormone can result giantism.

7. _____ Drug used for diabetes insipidus.

8. _____ Drug used to induce labor.

9. _____ Drug used in the treatment of infertility to induce ovulation.

10. _____ Drug used as a diagnostic test in suspected adrenal insufficiency.

11. _____ Sudden discontinuation of this drug may cause weakness, fatigue, and hypotension.

12. _____ Adverse effects of this drug include headache, nasal congestion, nausea, and hyponatremia.

A. Follicle-stimulating hormone (FSH).

B. Oxytocin (Pitocin).

C. Menotropins (Pergonal).

D. Melanocyte-stimulating hormone.

E. Cosyntropin (Cortrosyn).

F. Neurohypophysis.

G. Lypressin.

H. Antidiuretic hormone (ADH).

I. Prolactin.

J. Corticotropin (ACTH).

K. Desmopressin acetate (Stimate).

L. Growth hormone.

FILL IN THE BLANKS

Fill in the blanks in the chart with the terms listed below to describe pituitary function.

ACTH	Oxytocin	Growth hormone
FSH	TSH	LH
Prolactin	ADH	

Chart

Anterior Pituitary		**Posterior Pituitary**
1. _____ Stimulates secretion of milk	5. _____ **Female** Stimulates ovulation and luteinization **Male** Stimulates spermatogenesis	7. _____ Promotes retention of water (reduces urinary volume)
2. _____ Regulates body growth		8. _____ Contracts muscle in wall of uterus
3. _____ Regulates thyroid gland activity	6. _____ **Female** Stimulates growth and activity of ovarian follicles **Male** Stimulates growth of seminiferous tubules and spermatogenesis	
4. _____ Regulates activity of the adrenal cortex		

REVIEW QUESTIONS

1. Your client is being treated for adrenal dysfunction. You know that she understands the teaching you have done regarding corticotropin (ACTH) if she states the following:

   a. "I will not drink more than 1500 ml daily."

   b. "I will avoid excessive exposure to the sun."

   c. "I will weigh myself weekly and report a weight loss of more than 2 lb."

   d. "I will eat foods low in sodium and high in potassium."

2. You should contact the physician if you observe the following adverse effects during the administration of vasopressin (Pitressin):

   a. Bradycardia.

   b. Coughing.

   c. Chest pain.

   d. Diarrhea.

3. The nurse should instruct a client who is taking corticotropin (ACTH) that abrupt withdrawal of the drug can result in

   a. confusion, lethargy, and hypertension.

   b. nausea, vomiting, and diarrhea.

   c. headache, dizziness, and blurred vision.

   d. weakness, fatigue, and hypotension.

4. C.J. is receiving somatropin (Humatrope) because of a growth deficiency. Which of the following lab studies should be done on a regular basis?

   a. WBC.

   b. Serum glucose.

   c. Hemoglobin.

   d. Serum potassium levels.

5. Which of the following medications, if administered with vasopressin, would decrease its effect?

   a. Estrogen.

   b. Lithium carbonate (Eskalith).

   c. Cosyntropin (Cortrosyn).

   d. Chlorpropamide (Diabinese).

6. Which of the following medications, if administered concurrently with oxytocin (Pitocin), will produce hypertension?

   a. Estrogen.

   b. Ephedrine sulfate.

   c. Propranolol (Inderal).

   d. Atropine.

7. An expected outcome after administration of desmopressin (Stimate) is decreased

   a. blood pressure.

   b. serum potassium levels.

   c. specific gravity.

   d. urinary output.

8. Adverse effects that the nurse administering lypressin should assess for include

   a. chest pain.

   b. arrhythmias.

   c. hypotension.

   d. dyspnea.

9. Somatropin (Humatrope) should be administered to children with growth impairment before

   a. age 2.

   b. entering school.

   c. puberty.

   d. age 18.

CRITICAL THINKING CASE STUDY

Ms. G., an 18-year-old primigravida, has been in labor for 6 hours and her labor is not progressing. Her physician decides to start an oxytocin (Pitocin) drip.

1. Explain to Ms. G. the rationale for starting this medication and what she can expect.

2. Identify your nursing responsibilities.

The order for the oxytocin (Pitocin) reads: 1–2 milliunits/minute; increase by 1–2 milliunits every 15 minutes.

3. Discuss why the medication is administered in this way.

One hour after starting the oxytocin (Pitocin) Ms. G. starts screaming, "I can't take the pain; do something!"

4. Identify and prioritize your nursing actions.

Ms. G. delivers an 8 lb 8 oz healthy baby boy. After delivery, the physician wants the oxytocin (Pitocin) drip continued. Ms. G. starts crying and says, "Why can't they stop the medication now that I've had the baby?"

5. Identify your best response.

24

Corticosteroids

TRUE OR FALSE

1. _____ Secretion of corticosteroids normally decreases during periods of stress.

2. _____ Secretion of corticosteroids is normally controlled by a positive feedback mechanism.

3. _____ Endogenous corticosteroids are those obtained from a source outside the human body.

4. _____ Glucocorticoids promote wound healing.

5. _____ Glucocorticoids may cause hyperglycemia and diabetes mellitus as a result of increased production and decreased use of glucose.

6. _____ Glucocorticoids are often given therapeutically for anti-inflammatory effects.

7. _____ Aldosterone conserves water and sodium and eliminates potassium.

8. _____ Sex hormones are produced by the adrenal glands of both men and women.

9. _____ Corticosteroid drugs cure the diseases for which they are given.

10. _____ A major adverse effect of corticosteroid drug therapy is suppression of the HPA axis.

11. _____ Glucocorticoid therapy can precipitate gastrointestinal bleeding.

12. _____ Long-term corticosteroid drug therapy should be reserved for life-threatening conditions or severe, disabling symptoms that do not respond to other measures.

13. _____ The dosage of corticosteroids must be tapered slowly when the drug is discontinued.

14. _____ Alternate day therapy is used for children receiving corticosteroids so it does not affect their growth.

15. _____ When corticosteroids are being used for adrenal insufficiency, they should be administered between 6 P.M. and 9 P.M.

16. _____ Persons using corticosteroids may need potassium supplementation.

17. _____ Osteoporosis is an adverse effect of long-term corticosteroid therapy.

18. _____ Acne is effectively treated with steroids.

CHECKLIST

Undesirable Effects of Drug Administration

Place a check mark beside the words or phrases that indicate adverse effects of corticosteroid drug therapy.

1. _____ Dehydration.

2. _____ Rounded or "moon" face.

3. _____ Hyperglycemia.

4. _____ Delayed wound healing.

5. _____ Edema.

6. _____ Inhibition of bone growth.

7. _____ Oliguria.

8. _____ Protein depletion.

9. _____ Hypertension.

10. _____ Tissue wasting.

11. _____ Impaired ability to cope with stress.

12. _____ Euphoria.

13. _____ Cushing's disease.

14. _____ Hypernatremia.

15. _____ Hypercorticism.

16. _____ Nausea and vomiting.

17. _____ Change in sleep patterns.

18. _____ Diarrhea.

19. _____ Excessive sweating.

20. _____ Depression.

21. _____ Personality changes.

22. _____ Increased intraocular pressure.

23. _____ Anorexia.

24. _____ Peptic ulcer disease.

WORD SCRAMBLE

Provide the trade name for each generic name, then circle the trade name in the word find.

1. beclomethasone _____
2. betamethasone _____
3. fludrocortisone _____
4. flunisolide _____
5. triamcinolone
   hexacetonide _____
6. hydrocortisone _____
7. methylprednisolone _____
8. prednisolone _____
9. cortisone _____
10. dexamethasone _____
11. paramethasone _____
12. triamcinolone _____
13. prednisolone
    sodium phosphate _____
14. prednisone _____

REVIEW QUESTIONS

1. The corticosteroid of choice for treating cerebral edema is
   a. triamcinolone acetonide (Azmacort)
   b. betamethasone (Celestone).
   c. cortisone (Cortone).
   d. dexamethasone (Decadron).

2. Administration of corticosteroids causes
   a. sodium to be excreted.
   b. potassium to be excreted.
   c. potassium to be reabsorbed.
   d. hydrogen to be reabsorbed.

3. You are admitting 65-year-old Mr. J., who is to receive methylprednisolone sodium succinate (Solu Medrol) for asthma. For which of the following diseases should steroids be administered with caution?
   a. Peripheral vascular disease.
   b. Prostatic hypertrophy.
   c. Chronic obstructive pulmonary disease.
   d. Peptic ulcer disease.

Word Find

```
A P P L H E X N O T H S B H Y P O F T I L C L C E
B F G H D J K A D R E N E R G I C E N B E C T A Z
C O L A E N E C M R A I S S A N L L X Q K O V Z S
D E A N L V C D N C H T N H X Y Z T I P L R D N E
E G G H T D R O E O N I R Y L A R N V R H T L P O
F O N T A D I L N C A Y Y D O D A V P P J O F N V
A N L E S C B R E I K X F E H T G N A E B N O S B
R I F L O R I N E F L U A L A C A A I D A E U K L
O E E U N R E T O R P M X T T O S H R F R N O H A
Y P X C E L E S T O N E D R K B B L K A O T L R N
A J R E C L N O N O T D H A R I S T O C O R T S B
H Y P O F T I L C L C R E S F G H H J N K K A D R
E N E R G I C E L N B O E O T D A Z O L O L A N E
C M R A I S S I A N E L L L X E K V Z S X C W C A
H L P O D I R L A U D I D N A C A Y Y O D A U P J
R I L U A E A C A A I D A V H A L D R O N E H A P
D K B E C L A O T L R N A Y J D R E C L N O S T Y
M P E N A M B E R E C V A S G R O N I Q P P F E N
T A A E R O B I D N Y L K I G O N L O K C T K X T
G V A A N G A R I S T O S P A N T A P E S C O R N
I U O U S A L E T M O D T I I B T U D H T R P P L
A S O N B S O R P H Y D R O C O C O R T E F I O N
C W A C I N U C N K I X O P T O R I T A R N G I N
Y B P I X K U N L S I N E T A X A A Y B A I D L E
```

4. Your client is being treated with cortisone (Cortone). You know the drug is effective if there is a decrease in the symptoms of adrenal insufficiency, which include

   a. anxiety, restlessness, insomnia.

   b. diarrhea, tachycardia, hypertension.

   c. weakness, anorexia, hypotension.

   d. hyperglycemia, hypernatremia, hypokalemia.

5. Your client is a type II diabetic who is to be started on prednisone (Deltasone) for arthritis. You should be aware of the potential for

   a. decreased blood glucose levels.

   b. increased serum potassium levels.

   c. decreased effectiveness of prednisone.

   d. increased blood glucose levels.

6. You know that your client, who is taking cortisone acetate (Cortone) for arthritis, understands the discharge teaching you have done if he states

   a. "I will stop the medicine if I become drowsy."

   b. "I will use aspirin-containing products as needed."

   c. "I will take my medication with an antacid to prevent GI irritation."

   d. "I will have my blood pressure checked daily."

7. Which of the following medications, if administered with corticosteroids, will decrease their effect?

   a. Thiazide diuretics.

   b. Estrogens.

   c. Amitriptyline (Elavil).

   d. Phenytoin (Dilantin).

8. Which of the following medications, if administered with corticosteroids, will increase their effect?

   a. Salicylates.

   b. Antihistamines.

   c. Barbiturates.

   d. Anticholinergic agents.

9. Dosages of corticosteroids need to be reduced if the following condition is present.

   a. Adrenal insufficiency.

   b. Diarrhea.

   c. Hyperthyroidism.

   d. Hypoalbuminemia.

10. G.P., age 9, is receiving prednisone along with other immunosuppressants to prevent rejection of his newly transplanted kidney. It is important for you to give G.P.'s parents which of the following instructions?

    a. Stunting of growth can occur with long-term steroid use.

    b. Long-term steroid use can prevent development of secondary sexual characteristics.

    c. Long-term steroid use can cause weight loss.

    d. Alopecia can occur with long-term steroid use.

CRITICAL THINKING CASE STUDY

G., age 9, is started on prednisone for glomerulonephritis because he has begun spilling protein into his urine.

1. Identify the instructions you will give G.'s mother before he goes home.

G.'s mother asks you what she can expect as far as length of treatment, ongoing tests, etc.

2. Describe how you will respond to her questions.

You see G.'s mother 6 months later and she is crying. She states that G. has gained 15 lb and that the children at school are making fun of her son and he is very unhappy.

3. Identify the best response to K.'s mother, including any suggestions that would be helpful.

25

Thyroid and Antithyroid Drugs

FILL IN THE BLANKS

Complete the following sentences.

1. Production of T_3 and T_4 depends on the presence of _____.

2. Thyroid hormone controls _____.

3. Thyroid hormones are required for _____ and _____.

4. Symptoms of hypothyroidism in children include _____, _____, _____, _____, _____, and _____.

5. The symptoms of adult hypothyroidism or _____ are _____.

6. A person with hyperthyroidism will exhibit these CNS effects: _____, _____, _____, _____, _____, and _____.

7. Thyroid storm or thyrotoxic crisis is characterized by _____, _____, _____, and _____.

8. Hyperthyroidism is treated by _____, _____, _____, or _____.

9. The drug of choice for treating hypothyroidism is _____, and it is administered _____ per day. The usual maintenance dose is _____ mg daily.

10. Propylthiouracil (Propacil) is used to treat _____.

11. An antiadrenergic drug used to treat cardiovascular conditions associated with hyperthyroidism is _____ (_____).

12. The normal values for T_3 are _____ and for T_4 are _____.

13. Antithyroid drugs are administered for _____ months.

14. Children who are receiving thyroid replacement should have the following parameters monitored regularly: _____ and _____.

15. In older adults, levothyroxine (Synthroid) should be held if the resting HR is greater than _____.

NURSING DIAGNOSIS

S., age 5, is taken to the pediatrician for her school physical and hyperthyroidism is discovered. Identify three possible nursing diagnoses, pertinent assessment data, and nursing interventions associated with hyperthyroidism.

1. Nursing Diagnosis:

    Assessment Data:

    Nursing Interventions:

2. Nursing Diagnosis:

    Assessment Data:

    Nursing Interventions:

3. Nursing Diagnosis:

    Assessment Data:

    Nursing Interventions:

DEFINITIONS

Define the following terms.

1. Goiter

    _____

2. Cretinism

    _____

3. Myxedema

    _____

4. Thyroid storm

    _____

REVIEW QUESTIONS

1. After a thyroidectomy, your client is placed on Synthroid. Which of the following statements would indicate that your client has understood the teaching you have done?

    a. "I can expect to feel tired and nauseated initially."

    b. "I will monitor my weight and pulse regularly."

    c. "When my symptoms subside, I will no longer need medication."

    d. "I can continue to use over the counter cold preparations."

2. Mr. J. has blood work done. His T_3 is 0.08 and T4 is 10 mg/100 ml. From the results of the lab work, you know that his medication dose

    a. needs to be increased.

    b. needs to be decreased.

    c. needs to be discontinued.

    d. is adequate.

3. Mrs. P. is taking thyroid preparations for hypothyroidism. Which of the following would be indicative of an improvement in her condition?

    a. Normoactive reflexes.

    b. Weight gain.

    c. Long menstrual periods.

    d. Decreased appetite.

4. Which of the following diagnoses is appropriate for someone with hypothyroidism?

    a. Altered bowel elimination: diarrhea.

    b. Altered nutrition: less than body requirements.

    c. Risk for infection.

    d. Decreased cardiac output.

5. Children who are receiving thyroid replacement should have which of the following parameters monitored regularly?

    a. Urine specific gravity.

    b. Muscle mass.

    c. Intellectual development.

    d. Pulmonary function.

6. Which of the following drugs, when administered concurrently with thyroid hormones, increase their effects?

    a. Antidepressants.

    b. Beta-adrenergic blockers.

    c. Oral contraceptives.

    d. Antihypertensives.

7. Persons with hypothyroidism are especially sensitive to narcotics and sedatives and should be observed for the following when they are administered:

   a. Confusion.

   b. Tachycardia.

   c. Respiratory depression.

   d. Hypertension.

8. Persons taking propylthiouracil (Propacil) should be instructed about the adverse effects of the medication, which include

   a. tachycardia.

   b. blood dyscrasias.

   c. edema of the eyelids.

   d. hypertension.

9. Miss G., a 22-year-old, is to be started on a thyroid preparation. Which of the following questions is important to ask her before initiating treatment?

   a. "Have you ever had elevated blood pressure?"

   b. "Are you presently using birth control pills?"

   c. "Do you take aspirin on a regular basis?"

   d. "Do you have a history of respiratory problems?"

10. When assessing a client on thyroid replacement for hypothyroidism, you should monitor the client for

   a. hypertension.

   b. insomnia.

   c. bradycardia.

   d. weight gain.

CRITICAL THINKING CASE STUDY

Mrs. G, a 21-year-old female, has lost 10 lb since she was seen by her physician a year ago. She complains of headaches, insomnia, excessive perspiration, and palpitations. Her VS are BP 100/60, pulse 120, respirations 16. Her physician diagnoses her with hyperthyroidism and starts her on propylthiouracil (Propacil) and propranolol (Inderal).

1. Identify which of Mrs. G's signs and symptoms are attributable to hyperthyroidism?

2. Explain to Mrs. G. why her physician ordered propranolol (Inderal) and propylthiouracil (Propacil), how long she will need to take the medications, and when she can expect to see therapeutic effects from the medications.

3. Describe the instructions that you will give Mrs. G. regarding the adverse effects of the medications she is taking.

Two years after her initial treatment, Mrs. G. returns to the physician. She has gained 20 lb and complains of being tired. The physician orders thyroid function studies and finds the results to be below the normal range. He starts Mrs. G. on 0.125 mg of Synthroid.

4. Identify why hypothyroidism must be treated.

5. Describe the instructions you will give Mrs. G. regarding Synthroid.

26

Hormones That Regulate Calcium and Phosphorus Metabolism

FILL IN THE BLANKS

Complete the following sentences.

1. Calcium and phosphorus metabolism is regulated by _____ and _____, as well as vitamin D.

2. Generally, when serum calcium levels go _____, serum phosphate levels go _____.

3. When calcium levels are low, the effect of parathyroid hormone on the following tissues is
   a. Bone: _____
   b. Intestine: _____
   c. Kidneys: _____

4. Calcitonin _____ serum calcium levels by decreasing movement of calcium from _____ to _____.
   Its action is _____ but _____. It has little effect on _____ calcium metabolism.

5. Vitamin D is obtained from _____ and _____. The main action of vitamin D is to raise _____ by

_____ intestinal absorption of dietary calcium and _____.

6. Calcitriol (_____), a vitamin D preparation, is administered _____.

7. Deficiency of vitamin D causes inadequate absorption of _____ and _____.

8. The normal serum calcium level is _____.

9. Calcium is important in the regulation of
   a. _____
   b. _____
   c. _____
   d. _____
   e. _____
   f. _____

10. Sources of calcium include _____, _____, and _____.

11. Factors that inhibit calcium absorption include _____, _____, _____, _____, and _____.

12. Phosphorus in important because it
   a. _____
   b. _____
   c. _____
   d. _____
   e. _____

13. Clinical manifestations of hypocalcemia are characterized by increased _____, which may progress to _____.

14. Metabolic acidosis _____ the concentration of ionized calcium.

15. Two tests that help determine the presence of tetany are _____ sign and _____ sign.

16. A drug that increases the absorption of calcium is _____.

17. Injections of these drugs can cause hypercalcemia: _____, _____, _____, and _____.

18. Hypercalcemia has a _____ effect on nerve and muscle function.

19. Hypercalcemia can lead to calcium deposits in the kidneys, which may lead to _____ and _____.

20. Calcitonin-salmon (Calcimar) _____ serum calcium levels.

21. Furosemide (_____) _____ calcium excretion in urine by preventing its reabsorption in renal tubules.

22. Hydrocortisone and prednisone antagonize the effects of _____, thus _____ intestinal absorption of calcium.

23. Plicamycin (Mithracin) lowers serum calcium by _____.

24. Normal saline inhibits _____,

25. For clients experiencing hypercalcemia, fluids should be increased to _____ ml/day.

TRUE OR FALSE

1. ____ Women over 50 can benefit from calcium and vitamin D supplements.
2. ____ Administration of laxatives can cause hypercalcemia.
3. ____ If calcium is given to a digitalized client, the risks of digitalis toxicity increase.
4. ____ Persons receiving anticonvulsant therapy are likely to develop hypercalcemia.
5. ____ Oral calcium preparations should not be administered with tetracycline because they affect its absorption.

REVIEW QUESTIONS

1. Which of the following will cause decreased serum calcium levels?
   a. Prednisone (Deltasone).
   b. Calcitriol (Rocaltrol).
   c. Cholecalciferol (Delta-D).
   d. Dihydrotachysterol (Hytakerol).

2. Which of the following electrolyte imbalances will lower serum calcium levels?
   a. Hyperphosphatemia.
   b. High serum albumin levels.
   c. Low serum sodium levels.
   d. Hypokalemia.

3. When Mrs. J. is admitted to the hospital, a low serum calcium level is discovered. Which of the following might you expect Mrs. J. to complain of?
   a. Headache and dizziness.
   b. Drowsiness.
   c. Muscle flaccidity.
   d. Numbness and tingling in lips and hands.

4. Which statement would lead you to believe that your client understands the teaching that you have done regarding calcium supplements?
   a. "I will take the medication 30 minutes before meals or at bedtime."
   b. "I will take the calcium with antacids to prevent nausea."
   c. "I will contact my physician immediately if I become constipated."
   d. "I must limit my intake of foods high in vitamin K."

5. Your client is admitted with respiratory alkalosis. Which electrolyte imbalance should you assess for?
   a. Hypercalcemia.
   b. Hypocalcemia.
   c. Hypophosphatemia.
   d. Hyperkalemia.

6. Mrs. C. has a low serum calcium level. Which of the following foods should you recommend?
   a. Red meat.
   b. Whole grains.
   c. Dark green leafy vegetables.
   d. Citrus fruits.

7. Mrs. H. is experiencing acute hypercalcemia. The treatment of choice is

    a. phosphate salts (Neutra-Phos) and a high fruit intake.

    b. etidronate (Didronel) and D$_5$W.

    c. calcitonin-salmon (Calcimar) and lactated Ringers.

    d. furosemide (Lasix) and normal saline.

8. Mrs. D. is admitted with a serum calcium level of 12.5 mg/dl. You know that this is

    a. below the therapeutic range.

    b. within the therapeutic range.

    c. above the therapeutic range.

    d. extremely high.

9. Mrs. B., who is taking calcium, should avoid concurrent use of the following because it decreases the effects of calcium:

    a. Alcohol.

    b. Vitamin D.

    c. Bran.

    d. Laxatives.

10. Miss J. is taking calcium supplements, and her physician starts her on tetracycline. Which of the following instructions should she receive?

    a. "Take these medications with meals."

    b. "Take both medications on an empty stomach."

    c. "Take tetracycline an hour before meals and calcium with meals."

    d. "Take medications three hours apart."

CRITICAL THINKING CASE STUDY

J.C. is admitted to your unit in acute renal failure, with the following lab values: creatinine 3.8, calcium 12.8 mg/100 ml, potassium 6.8. The physician orders furosemide (Lasix) 40 mg IV, hydrocortisone (Solu Cortef) 40 mg IV, and 1000 cc 0.9% NaCl to run at 50 cc/hour. (The learner will need additional sources to answer the questions.)

1. Identify what you will be assessing for when J.C. is admitted.

2. Discuss the rationale for the treatment plan.

A dual lumen catheter is inserted and J.C. is dialyzed. When J.C. returns from dialysis, he complains of a headache and nausea.

3. Identify what you will do next.

J.C. is to continue to take furosemide (Lasix) once he returns home.

4. Identify the teaching that you will do with J.C. and his mother to prepare them for discharge.

27

Antidiabetic Agents

FILL IN THE BLANKS

Use the following terms to fill in the blanks.

increases   decreases

1. Insulin
   a. _____ storage of glycogen and fatty acids.
   b. _____ the breakdown of glucose.
   c. _____ protein breakdown.
   d. _____ protein and glycogen synthesis.
   e. _____ production of glycerol and fatty acids
   f. _____ breakdown of fats.
   g. _____ blood glucose levels.

MATCHING EXERCISE

Terms and Concepts

Match the concept with the term for it.

1. _____ A type of hyperglycemia that occurs following an insulin-induced hypoglycemia reaction.

2. _____ Changes in fatty subcutaneous tissue occurring from frequent injections.

3. _____ Persons requiring large doses of insulin, possibly due to the development of antibodies.

4. _____ Symptoms include tachycardia, blurred vision, weakness, fatigue, and sweating.

5. _____ This drug increases the effects of oral agents.

6. _____ This drug raises blood glucose levels and antagonizes the effects of insulin.

7. _____ The normal range for blood glucose levels.

8. _____ Regular insulin peaks.

9. _____ This test reflects the average blood sugar for 2–3 months.

10. _____ A common complication that persons with diabetes experience.

A. Hyperglycemia.

B. MAO inhibitors.

C. Somogyi effect.

D. Lipodystrophy.

E. Allopurinol (Zyloprim).

F. Insulin resistance.

G. 80–120 mg/100 ml.

H. Hypoglycemia.

I. Oral contraceptives.

J. 60–100 mg/100 ml.

K. 2–3 hours.

L. 4–6 hours.

M. Glycosylated hemoglobin.

N. Urinary tract infections.

CROSSWORD PUZZLE

Across

5. A second-generation sulfonylurea, recommended for patients with impaired renal function.

7. One of the preferred types of insulin for long-term therapy.

8. This oral antidiabetic drug has a diuretic effect.

10. These drugs with insulin can increase the chance of hypoglycemia.

12. This reaction to insulin includes tachycardia, hunger, muscle tremors, and blurred vision.

Down

1. This type of insulin is preferred for poorly controlled diabetes.

2. Isotonic IV fluids are an important part of treating diabetic _____.

3. A useful drug for diabetics who have fluid retention and edema.

4. Preferred oral hypoglycemic for diabetics with gout.

6. Failing to change insulin injection sites can lead to this.

9. Lack of insulin leads to high blood _____ levels.

11. Insulin from this source is the most antigenic type.

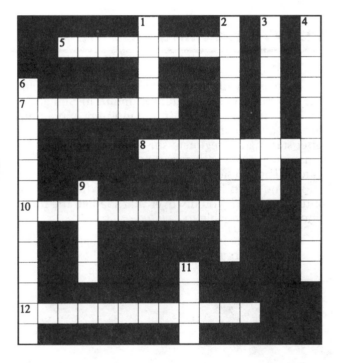

TRUE OR FALSE

1. _____ Early symptoms of diabetic ketoacidosis include blurred vision, anorexia, nausea, vomiting, thirst, and polyuria.

2. _____ Insulin can be stored at room temperature.

3. _____ Type II diabetics require only oral agents to control their diabetes mellitus.

4. _____ Oral agents are contraindicated during pregnancy.

5. _____ Once insulin has been started, the person will remain on the medication for the rest of his or her life.

6. _____ Symptoms of hypoglycemia include excessive thirst, hunger, and increased urine output.

7. _____ Salicylates taken with antidiabetic drugs increase the likelihood of hypoglycemia.

8. _____ Persons taking adrenocorticosteroids and thiazide diuretics will require less insulin.

9. _____ Insulin is necessary for normal growth and development in children.

10. _____ When treating hypoglycemia, the primary goal is to restore the brain's supply of glucose.

11. _____ A honeymoon period, characterized by recovery of islet function and temporary production of insulin, may occur after diabetes is first diagnosed and treated.

12. _____ Once hypoglycemia is relieved, the client should consume foods high in fat to replace glycogen stores and prevent secondary hypoglycemia.

13. _____ A diabetic may take both oral agents and insulin.

REVIEW QUESTIONS

1. Mr. J. is receiving short and long acting insulin in the morning. The most likely time of occurrence for hypoglycemic reactions is

   a. 10 A.M. and 4 P.M.

   b. 8 A.M. and 4 P.M.

   c. 11 A.M. and 6 P.M.

   d. 11 A.M. and 3 P.M.

2. Which of the following instructions should be given to a person who is taking insulin?

   a. Draw up NPH insulin first, then regular insulin.

   b. Inject insulin at a 45-degree angle in the subcutaneous tissue.

   c. Shake the NPH insulin thoroughly before administering it.

   d. Rotate injection sites; use upper back and buttock as well as arms, thighs, and abdomen.

3. Which of the following statements by your client leads you to believe that he needs additional teaching about diabetes?

   a. "I will weigh myself weekly and try to maintain my present weight."

   b. "After I begin feeling shaky, I have about 15 minutes before my blood sugar drops dangerously low."

   c. "I will test my blood sugar before and after I exercise."

   d. "I will avoid alcohol and concentrated sweets."

4. Prolonged hypoglycemia resulting from the administration of insulin can result in

   a. kidney damage.

   b. brain damage.

   c. hypoxia.

   d. hypotension.

5. A type II non-insulin-dependent diabetic may require insulin as a result of all of the following except

   a. surgery.

   b. pregnancy.

   c. infection.

   d. weight loss.

6. Mrs. J. is a type II diabetic who has recently been placed on insulin. Which of the following statements by Mrs. J. leads you to believe that she has understood the teaching that you have done?

   a. "I must take shots now because the oral insulin is no longer effective."

   b. "I know I must keep insulin refrigerated."

   c. "Human insulin is derived from human pancreas."

   d. "I will make sure the insulin I inject is not cold."

7. Administration of which of the following drugs can result in drug-induced diabetes mellitus?

   a. Antidiabetic agents.

   b. Beta-adrenergic blockers.

   c. Corticosteroids.

   d. Thiazide diuretics.

8. Mr. J.'s blood glucose comes back as 130 mg/100 ml. This value is

   a. below the normal range.

   b. within the normal range.

   c. above the normal range.

   d. extremely high.

9. When teaching J. about the signs and symptoms of hyperglycemia, you tell him he may experience

   a. sweating.

   b. polyuria.

   c. weakness.

   d. dizziness.

10. Which of the following statements is false?

    a. Weight loss will decrease insulin needs in diabetics.

    b. Oral agents and insulin cannot be used together.

    c. Regular insulin is the only type of insulin that may be given intravenously.

    d. Insulin pumps use buffered insulin.

CRITICAL THINKING CASE STUDY

Mrs. J. is newly diagnosed with type I diabetes mellitus. She takes 3 units Regular Humulin Insulin and 14 NPH Humulin Insulin in the morning and 6 units Regular and 10 units NPH before dinner. One month after starting the regimen, she is brought to the emergency room with sweating, tremor, and tachycardia. The physician diagnoses her with insulin shock and starts intravenous glucose. When you interview Mrs. J. you discover that she had the flu and had been unable to eat.

1. Identify the information you will share with Mrs. J. and her husband about diet and lifestyle changes to help her control her diabetes.

Mrs. J. calls her physician because she is having frequent hypoglycemia reactions in the middle of the night.

2. Identify what information you will discuss with Mrs. J. that will help her manage her hypoglycemia.

Mrs. J.'s physician changes her insulin to 3 units Regular Insulin and 4 units NPH in the morning, 6 units Regular Insulin at dinnertime, and 10 units of NPH at h.s.

4. Discuss why these changes were made.

Mr. J. calls the emergency room and states that his wife is unresponsive and asks you what to do.

3. Discuss your response to Mr. J.

28

Estrogen, Progestins, and Oral Contraceptives

14. _____ Birth control pills may only be taken for 5 years.

15. _____ Progestins reduce the risk of endometrial cancer in women.

FILL IN THE BLANKS

Complete the following sentence.

1. Estrogen is administered in postmenopausal women to prevent

   a. _____

   b. _____

   c. _____

   d. _____

NAME THAT DRUG

1. _____ Administered via patch, worn three consecutive weeks a month.

2. _____ Used topically for atrophic or senile vaginitis.

3. _____ Administered twice a day for 5 days for postcoital contraception.

4. _____ Can be administered intravenously for dysfunctional uterine bleeding.

5. _____ Administered intramuscularly at the end of the first stage of labor to prevent postpartum breast engorgement.

6. _____ Given intramuscularly in doses of 1.5–2 mg once a month to treat female hypogonadism.

7. _____ Given intramuscularly once every 4 weeks for four doses to treat amenorrhea or dysfunctional bleeding.

8. _____ Used for endometrial cancer, administered intramuscularly weekly until improvement, then monthly.

9. _____ A commonly prescribed estrogen used for treatment of menopause.

10. _____ This drug is used to prevent osteoporosis in postmenopausal women.

11. _____ This drug decreases the effects of oral anticoagulants, insulin, oral antidiabetic agents, and antihypertensive drugs.

TRUE OR FALSE

1. _____ The use of estrogen may aggravate gallbladder disease.

2. _____ Persons taking estrogen will need phosphorus supplementation.

3. _____ Progesterone stimulates milk production.

4. _____ Estrogen has been used to prevent excessive height in young girls.

5. _____ During pregnancy the placenta produces large amounts of estrogen.

6. _____ One of the problems associated with exogenous estrogen is dehydration.

7. _____ Progesterone decreases gastrointestinal motility.

8. _____ Women with diabetes mellitus may not use birth control pills.

9. _____ Diethylstilbestrol (Stilbestrol) is approved as a postcoital contraceptive.

10. _____ Estrogen and progestins should be taken on an empty stomach.

11. _____ Birth control pills are used in the treatment of amenorrhea.

12. _____ Estrogen may be administered after delivery to suppress lactation.

13. _____ Acne is a common adverse effect of taking birth control pills.

12. _____ This drug is used to treat ovarian failure.

13. _____ This drug is used to test estrogen production.

14. _____ An oral contraceptive that contains no estrogen.

15. _____ If this aminoglycoside is administered with oral contraceptives, it will decrease their effectiveness.

REVIEW QUESTIONS

1. Persons using birth control pills need to be assessed regularly for
   a. increased intraocular pressure.
   b. decreased urinary output.
   c. bradycardia.
   d. hypertension.

2. Mr. B., a 76-year-old male, is started on estrogen for metastatic prostatic cancer. Which of the following statements by Mr. B. leads you to believe he has understood the teaching that you have done?
   a. "I will take the medication on an empty stomach."
   b. "I may experience impotence, which will subside when the drug is stopped."
   c. "If my breasts become enlarged I will apply ice to them."
   d. "I will take this medication for the rest of my life."

3. Mrs. K. is a 34-year-old mother of two with a history of diabetes and cancer of the breast. She is on a low-residue diet for colitis. Which of the factors in Mrs. K.'s history would contraindicate the use of birth control pills?
   a. Cancer of the breast.
   b. Age.
   c. Diabetes.
   d. Colitis.

4. Estropipate (Ogen) is administered to women for
   a. atrophic vaginitis.
   b. dysfunctional uterine bleeding.
   c. osteoporosis.
   d. uterine cancer.

5. Which of the following medications is administered for treatment of prostatic cancer?
   a. Estropipate (Ogen).
   b. Medroxyprogesterone acetate (Depo-Provera).
   c. Estradiol cypionate (Depo-Estradiol).
   d. Polyestradiol phosphate (Estradurin).

6. Which of the following statements indicates that your client needs additional teaching about birth control pills?
   a. "I will monitor my weight and have my blood pressure checked monthly."
   b. "I may gain weight while I am taking these pills."
   c. "I will elevate my legs and take aspirin if I experience leg pain."
   d. "I know nausea is common but it should subside in a few weeks."

7. The following instructions should be included before estrone (Theelin) is started for dysfunctional uterine bleeding. You will take the medication
   a. daily until the bleeding is controlled, followed by progestin for 1 week.
   b. twice a day until the bleeding subsides, followed by a week of prophylactic therapy.
   c. three times a day until the bleeding stops.
   d. intramuscularly daily until the bleeding stops, followed by 2 weeks of the oral preparation.

8. Which of the following statements by Mrs. G. leads you to believe that she has a good understanding of how to treat postpartum breast engorgement?
   a. "I will take the Tylenol twice a day for 2 weeks."
   b. "I will take the aspirin q6h for six doses."
   c. "I should decrease my fluid intake."
   d. "If I experience swelling, I should go to the emergency room immediately."

9. Which of the following medications, when administered concurrently with oral contraceptives, will decrease their effect?
   a. Antimicrobials.
   b. Antihypertensives.
   c. Anticoagulants.
   d. Diabetic agents.

10. Miss G. has female hypogonadism and is being treated with estrogen. Which of the following statements leads you to believe that she has a good understanding about the medication?

   a. "I need to eat foods high in fiber."

   b. "I will weigh myself daily and call the doctor if I lose weight."

   c. "I will take the medication for the rest of my life."

   d. "I may experience breast enlargement or growth of hair in the pubic area."

CRITICAL THINKING CASE STUDY

Ms. G. has come to the gynecologist requesting birth control pills.

1. Identify what factors would contraindicate the use of birth control pills and why.

2. Identify the assessments that should be done before birth control is started.

Ms. G. calls you, after taking birth control pills for 2 months, stating that she has severe acne and has gained 5 pounds.

3. Identify your response to Ms. G.

29

Androgens and Anabolic Steroids

CIRCLE THE CORRECT ANSWER

1. There will be a(an) increase/decrease in skin thickness when androgens or anabolic steroids are administered.

2. With the administration of androgens or anabolic steroids, protein anabolism increases/decreases and protein catabolism increases/decreases.

3. When anabolic steroids are administered, there is a(an) increased/decreased secretion of FSH.

4. Administration of anabolic steroids to women increases/decreases the lining of the uterus.

5. Persons taking androgens or anabolic steroids will notice a(an) increase/decrease in muscle mass.

6. When androgens are administered to young children, the result will be a significant increase/decrease in growth.

7. Androgens increase/decrease the development of female sexual characteristics.

8. When androgens or anabolic steroids are administered, there will be a(an) increase/decrease in body weight.

9. Large amounts of anabolic steroids ingested by adult males can cause a(an) increased/decreased sperm count.

10. Androgens or anabolic steroids will increase/decrease appetite.

11. Administration of androgens or anabolic steroids results in a(an) increase/decrease in sodium and water retention.

12. Administration of anabolic steroids increases/decreases the risk of developing prostatic cancer.

13. Antihistamines taken with anabolic steroids will increase/decrease the effect of the steroids.

14. Persons taking anabolic steroids have documented a(an) increase/decrease in body hair.

15. Androgens or anabolic steroids increase/decrease hematocrit and hemoglobin levels.

16. Androgens increase/decrease epiphyseal closure in children.

17. High doses of anabolic steroids increase/decrease/have no effect on the incidence of adverse reactions.

18. Androgens increase/decrease the effect of insulin.

19. Androgens can increase/decrease blood pressure in the elderly.

20. Androgens can increase/decrease the size of the prostate gland.

CROSSWORD PUZZLE

Across

2. This drug's dosage may need to be decreased during androgen treatment.

3. One dangerous side effect of anabolic steroid use is an _____ imbalance.

5. Androgen therapy in children can lead to premature _____ closure.

6. For short-term treatment of postpartum breast engorgement.

7. Administered to younger males with cryptorchidism.

8. A hormone that stimulates testosterone secretion.

9. Used in the treatment of osteoporosis.

Down

1. Used to treat endometriosis and fibrocystic breast disease.

3. This type of androgen may be given orally.

4. Produced in the human body by Leydig's cells.

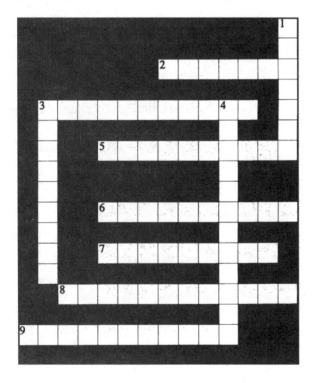

REVIEW QUESTIONS

1. Which of the following medications, if administered concurrently with anabolic steroids, will decrease their effect?
   a. Calcium channel blockers.
   b. Barbiturates.
   c. Thiazide diuretics.
   d. Anticholinergic drugs.

2. Persons taking anabolic steroids may experience which of the following beneficial effects?
   a. Increased muscle mass.
   b. Decreased appetite.
   c. Increased secretion of FSH and LH.
   d. Decreased serum sodium levels.

3. Physical changes that occur with the use of anabolic steroids in women include
   a. thinning of skin.
   b. increased menstrual flow.
   c. increased distribution of hair on body.
   d. increased endurance.

4. When androgens are administered to older adult males, the following can result:
   a. Gynecomastia.
   b. Rapid bone growth.
   c. Loss of pubic hair.
   d. Prostatic enlargement.

5. When nandrolone decanoate (Deca-Durabolin) is administered, an expected outcome is increased
   a. RBC production.
   b. serum albumin levels.
   c. serum potassium level.
   d. sperm count.

6. Mrs. A. is receiving methyltestosterone (Metandren) for advanced breast cancer. Which of the following should she have checked regularly?
   a. Renal function.
   b. Pulse rate.
   c. Hematocrit and hemoglobin.
   d. Liver function.

7. When nandrolone phenpropionate (Durabolin) is ordered for the treatment of anemia, it can cause
   a. hyperkalemia.
   b. osteoporosis.
   c. hypotension.
   d. sodium and water retention.

8. Mrs. H. is receiving nandrolone phenpropionate (Durabolin) for breast cancer. An adverse reaction resulting from the administration of this medication that the nurse needs to assess for is

   a. hypocalcemia.

   b. jaundice.

   c. skin rash.

   d. oliguria.

9. Androgens can potentiate the effect of oral antidiabetic agents. The dose of the oral antidiabetic drugs may need to be

   a. decreased.

   b. increased.

   c. stopped.

   d. changed to insulin.

10. Testosterone (Oreton) is ordered for B.J., age 11, who is experiencing hypogonadism. Which of the following statements by B.J. leads you to believe that he has understood the teaching that you have done regarding the medication?

    a. "I may experience visual changes as a result of taking this drug."

    b. "I will need to see the doctor every 6 months for x-rays."

    c. "If I experience acne, the drug will need to be stopped."

    d. "I can expect to lose weight as a result of taking this drug."

CRITICAL THINKING CASE STUDY

You are the school nurse at East Side High School. The wrestling coach asks you to give a presentation on anabolic steroids.

1. Develop a presentation that would convince teenage boys not to use anabolic steroids.

2. Identify ways the school nurse can monitor the health of high school athletes and possibly detect the use of steroids.

V

NUTRIENTS, FLUIDS, AND ELECTROLYTES

30

Nutritional Products, Anorexiants, and Digestants

FILL IN THE BLANKS

*Place a **P** for protein, a **C** for carbohydrate, a **W** for water, or an **F** for fat next to each body function. More than one nutrient may be listed for each body function.*

1. _____ Furnishes amino acids.

2. _____ Helps maintain body temperature.

3. _____ Promotes normal function of nerve cells.

4. _____ Assists in maintaining normal osmotic pressure.

5. _____ Transports nutrients to body cells.

6. _____ Promotes normal fat metabolism.

7. _____ Helps maintain electrolyte balance.

8. _____ Promotes bowel elimination.

9. _____ Protects organs from injury.

10. _____ Promotes normal growth and development.

TRUE OR FALSE

1. _____ An increased hematocrit is indicative of fluid volume excess.

2. _____ Persons with a water excess may experience disorientation.

3. _____ Persons with a protein deficit will be in metabolic alkalosis.

4. _____ Persons with a poor protein intake may have edema.

5. _____ Persons who are obese are more susceptible to developing an infection than undernourished persons.

6. _____ Some tube feedings are better tolerated if they are diluted initially.

7. _____ Intermittent feedings are preferable because diarrhea and gastric distention are decreased.

8. _____ A nasogastric tube will prevent the complication of aspiration.

9. _____ Pancreatic enzymes should be administered with food.

10. _____ Cold tube feedings are better tolerated than those at room temperature.

MATCHING EXERCISE

Match the formula or elemental diet with the population for which it is intended.

1. _____ Portagen.

2. _____ Pulmocare.

3. _____ Nutramigen.

4. _____ Flexical.

5. _____ Isomil.

6. _____ Pregestimil.

7. _____ Vivonex.

8. _____ Lofenalac.

9. _____ TraumaCal.

10. _____ Pediasure.

A. Infants with malabsorption syndromes.

B. Persons with chronic obstructive pulmonary disease.

C. Persons with fat and malabsorption problems.

D. Persons with GI disorders, because it requires no digestion and leaves no fecal residue.

E. Persons allergic to milk.

F. Children who are allergic to ordinary proteins.

G. Persons who have had bowel surgery.

H. Children ages 1–6.

I. Burn injury victims.

J. Children with phenylketonuria.

FILL IN THE BLANKS

Complete the following sentences.

1. The most commonly used dextrose solution is
   _____ and provides
   _____ kcal/liter.

2. For total parenteral nutrition,
   _____ and
   _____ solutions are used. They
   are _____, so they must be
   given through a central line.

3. Five hundred milliliters of a 10% fat emulsion
   provides _____ calories.

4. When a person is receiving tube feedings, additional _____ is necessary
   between feedings.

5. Most tube feedings are _____
   and will therefore _____ the
   fluid volume deficit if water is not administered
   with them.

6. TPN or hyperalimentation contains
   _____ and
   _____.

7. Fat emulsions provide _____
   and can be administered _____
   or _____.

8. Before administering a tube feeding, the nurse
   should check _____.

9. The maximum amount, including water, that
   should be administered at any one time is
   _____.

10. Clients receiving 2000 cc/day of tube feeding
    daily should receive _____ ml
    of water.

REVIEW QUESTIONS

1. 500 ml of a 10% fat emulsion provides
   a. 170 calories.
   b. 220 calories.
   c. 300 calories.
   d. 550 calories.

2. 1000 ml of $D_{10}W$ provides
   a. 340 calories.
   b. 480 calories.
   c. 550 calories.
   d. 1000 calories.

3. The following medication, if administered concurrently with anorexiants, will decrease their effect:
   a. Sodium bicarbonate.
   b. Tricyclic antidepressants.
   c. Vitamin C.
   d. Epinephrine.

4. Which of the following liquid formulas is the
   most appropriate for a baby who has diarrhea or
   a malabsorption syndrome?
   a. Portagen.
   b. Pediasure.
   c. Pregestimil.
   d. Lofenalac.

5. Persons receiving anorexiant drugs that contain
   phenylpropanolamine should be instructed about
   the adverse effects, which include
   a. hepatotoxicity.
   b. weakness, dizziness, and blurred vision.
   c. renal failure.
   d. nausea, vomiting, and diarrhea.

6. Persons receiving TPN (total parenteral nutrition)
   should be observed for
   a. a fluid deficit and metabolic acidosis.
   b. increased urinary output.
   c. elevated blood glucose levels.
   d. lower serum sodium levels.

7. A physician has ordered Polycose for M.J., a burn
   victim, because it
   a. is a high-protein substance, which M.J. needs
      right now.
   b. supplies a concentrated source of calories,
      protein, and electrolytes.
   c. is an additive that is mixed with food or bev-
      erages to increase the caloric intake.
   d. is an oral supplement that will increase M.J.'s
      protein, vitamin, and mineral intake.

8. Mr. P. is receiving a fat emulsion and begins complaining of dyspnea and chest pain. Identify what your first nursing action should be.

   a. Slow down the rate of the infusion.

   b. Check Mr. P.'s vital signs.

   c. Contact Mr. P.'s physician.

   d. Stop the fat emulsion infusion.

9. Your client, who has a 10-year history of chronic renal failure, is to receive Amin Aid for his supplemental feedings because

   a. it supplies amino acids, carbohydrates, and few electrolytes.

   b. its metabolism produces less carbon dioxide.

   c. it is high in nitrogen and high in carbohydrates.

   d. it requires no digestion and leaves no fecal residue.

10. Mrs. J., who is admitted with severe dehydration, will have a(n)

    a. elevated hematocrit.

    b. low serum sodium.

    c. protein deficit.

    d. low serum potassium.

CRITICAL THINKING CASE STUDY

Mr. J. is a 76-year-old man with a 10-year history of COPD. His most recent hospital admission is for a CVA. He is unresponsive and has a large pressure sore on his coccyx. A nasogastric tube is inserted and he is to receive 80 ml of Pulmocare and 40 ml of H_2O per hour in continuous feedings.

1. Identify why Pulmocare was chosen for the supplemental feeding for Mr. J.

2. Identify the nursing assessment that you will do for Mr. J.

3. Discuss the advantages and disadvantages of TPN and internal feedings and identify why Mr. J. was started on tube feeding instead of TPN.

4. Identify potential problems that a client with a tube feeding can experience and how these problems can be avoided.

Mr. J. experiences diarrhea four times during your shift.

5. Identify your nursing actions.

31

Vitamins

E. Pantothenic acid (vitamin B_5).

F. Vitamin E.

G. Thiamine (vitamin B_1).

H. Vitamin K.

I. Pyridoxine (vitamin B_6).

J. Biotin.

K. Vitamin D.

L. Cyanocobalamin (vitamin B_{12}).

M. Vitamin C (ascorbic acid).

NAME THAT DEFICIENCY/EXCESS

*Specify a vitamin and **deficiency** or **excess** for each condition. More than one vitamin may relate to a condition.*

1. _____ Causes night blindness.

2. _____ Results in bleeding abnormalities.

3. _____ Symptoms include anorexia, nausea, depression, and muscle pain.

4. _____ Causes convulsions, peripheral neuritis, and mental depression.

5. _____ Can cause renal calculi.

6. _____ Causes Wernicke–Korsakoff syndrome.

7. _____ Neurologic symptoms of this disorder include paresthesia, unsteady gait, and depressed deep tendon reflexes.

8. _____ Can cause scurvy.

9. _____ Causes impaired growth in children.

10. _____ Increases intracranial pressure.

11. _____ May be caused by smoking.

12. _____ Causes eye disorders (burning, itching, photophobia).

13. _____ Causes delusions, hallucinations, and impaired peripheral motor function.

14. _____ Can increase the amounts of oxalate in urine.

15. _____ Causes pernicious anemia.

16. _____ Results from a lack of hydrochloric acid or intrinsic factor in the stomach.

MATCHING EXERCISE

Terms and Concepts

Match the concept with the term for it.

1. _____ Required for normal vision.

2. _____ Found in cereals, green vegetables, egg yolk, and vegetable oils.

3. _____ Essential for normal clotting.

4. _____ Essential in fat and carbohydrate metabolism.

5. _____ Necessary for the normal development of RBCs and for growth.

6. _____ Found in liver, kidney beans, and green vegetables.

7. _____ Essential for fat synthesis.

8. _____ Necessary for the synthesis of cholesterol.

9. _____ Helps maintain cellular immunity.

10. _____ May function in production of corticosteroids and RBCs and in gluconeogenesis.

11. _____ Found in dried beans, whole grains, and peanuts.

12. _____ Not stored in body to a significant extent; excess excreted in the urine.

13. _____ Fat-soluble vitamin obtained from exposure of skin to sunlight.

A. Folic acid (folate).

B. Niacin (vitamin B_3).

C. Riboflavin (vitamin B_2).

D. Vitamin A.

17. _____ Occurs commonly in newborns.

18. _____ Early manifestations include anorexia, vomiting, irritability, and skin changes.

19. _____ Alcoholism is a common cause.

20. _____ Persons using oral contraceptives are at risk for developing this.

REVIEW QUESTIONS

1. Which of the following is a fat-soluble vitamin that may cause toxicity?
   a. Vitamin A.
   b. Vitamin B_6.
   c. Vitamin C.
   d. Folic acid (Folvite).

2. The adverse effects of administering large amounts of vitamin C include development of
   a. skin rashes.
   b. kidney stones.
   c. constipation.
   d. elevated uric acid levels.

3. A vitamin deficiency commonly found in alcoholics that is treated with vitamin supplementation is
   a. pantothenic acid (vitamin B_5) deficiency.
   b. vitamin A deficiency.
   c. vitamin D deficiency.
   d. thiamine (vitamin B_1) deficiency.

4. An expected outcome of the administration of vitamin B_{12} is
   a. decreased appetite.
   b. increased strength.
   c. decreased joint pain.
   d. improved vision.

5. The antidote for warfarin (Coumadin) is
   a. vitamin A.
   b. vitamin B_{12}.
   c. vitamin E.
   d. vitamin K.

6. Mr. J., a homeless man, is found by the side of the road. He is delusional and having auditory and visual hallucinations. His symptoms may be attributed to the following vitamin deficiency:
   a. Ascorbic acid (vitamin C).
   b. Riboflavin (vitamin B_1).
   c. Pantothenic acid (vitamin B_5).
   d. Niacin (vitamin B_3).

7. Mrs. H. is experiencing fatigue, anorexia, depression, and irritability. A deficiency of which of these vitamins can cause these symptoms?
   a. Vitamin A.
   b. Vitamin B_{12}.
   c. Vitamin C.
   d. Vitamin B_1.

8. Which of the following statements by your client leads you to believe she has understood the teaching that you have done regarding vitamin B_{12}?
   a. "The intrinsic factor in my stomach that is required for absorption of vitamin B_{12} is absent, so I must take shots."
   b. "Long-term use of this drug is associated with peripheral neuropathies."
   c. "Pernicious anemia causes changes in the mucous membrane lining and impairs absorption, so I may have diarrhea once I start this drug."
   d. "I will take this medication for a few months until I feel better."

9. A vitamin administered for treatment of hyperlipidemia is
   a. Pyridoxine (vitamin B_6).
   b. Pantothenic acid (vitamin B_5).
   c. Niacin (vitamin B_3).
   d. Riboflavin (vitamin B_2).

10. Before administering vitamin B_{12}, the following test(s) should be performed to determine the presence of pernicious anemia:
    a. Hematocrit and hemoglobin.
    b. Shick test.
    c. Sweat test.
    d. Shilling test.

CRITICAL THINKING CASE STUDY

Mr. B., a severely malnourished 56-year-old alcoholic, is admitted to your unit. Mr. B.'s physician orders niacin (vitamin B_3), thiamine (vitamin B_1), and folic acid (folate).

1. Specify the nursing assessments that you will do (including analysis of lab studies) when Mr. J. is admitted.

2. Discuss the rationale for using these medications and why they are administered parenterally.

Two days after admission, Mr. B. states, "I will not take any more shots and that is final."

3. Discuss how you will proceed.

32

Minerals and Electrolytes

MATCHING EXERCISE

Terms and Concepts

Match the concept with the term for it.

1. _____ Necessary for normal cell growth and synthesis of carbohydrates and proteins.

2. _____ Essential component of hemoglobin.

3. _____ Causes skeletal muscle weakness, respiratory insufficiency, and drowsiness.

4. _____ Causes abdominal distension, constipation, and paralytic ileus.

5. _____ This trace element is found in seafood.

6. _____ Strengthens bones by promoting calcium retention.

7. _____ This trace element is found in brain, heart, liver, kidneys, bone, and muscle.

8. _____ A component of vitamin B_{12} that is required for normal function of all body cells.

9. _____ Symptoms include headache, dizziness, weakness, lethargy, restlessness, confusion, convulsions.

10. _____ An exchange resin used for the treatment of hyperkalemia.

11. _____ A chelating agent used to remove excess iron.

12. _____ Increases the effectiveness of insulin.

13. _____ Assists in regulating osmotic pressure.

14. _____ Eliminated from the body primarily by the kidneys.

15. _____ Shifts in and out of the red blood cells in exchange for bicarbonate.

A. Copper.

B. Hyponatremia.

C. Deferoxamine (Desferal mesylate).

D. Hypermagnesemia.

E. Chromium.

F. Iron.

G. Zinc.

H. Hypokalemia.

I. Fluoride.

J. Sodium.

K. Cobalt.

L. Potassium.

M. Iodine.

N. Magnesium.

O. Chloride.

P. Sodium polystyrene sulfonate (Kayexalate).

NAME THAT IMBALANCE

Specify the imbalance associated with each condition. More than one imbalance may relate to a condition.

1. _____ Causes peaked T waves, prolonged P-R intervals, and prolonged QRS complexes.

2. _____ Signs and symptoms include impaired growth, anorexia, loss of taste and smell, and poor wound healing.

3. _____ Results in increased extracellular volume.

4. _____ Occurs in women who take oral contraceptives.

5. _____ Can occur as a result of acidosis.

6. _____ Produces impaired glucose tolerance and impaired growth and reproduction.

7. _____ Causes depressed ST segments and inverted T waves.

8. _____ Menke's syndrome is caused by this.

9. _____ Hypotension is a symptom of this.

10. _____ Results in bronze pigmentation of the skin.

11. _____ Hyperaldosteronism and Cushing's disease can cause this.

12. _____ Results in impaired erythropoiesis.

13. _____ Can result in overhydration and swelling of brain cells.

14. _____ Results in skeletal muscle weakness and paralysis.

15. _____ Impairs carbohydrate metabolism and decreases secretion of insulin.

16. _____ Excessive administration of ammonium chloride can cause this.

17. _____ Muscle spasms and tetany can result from this.

18. _____ Administration of large amounts of penicillin G can cause this.

19. _____ Commonly occurs with alcoholism.

20. _____ Causes depressant effects on the neuromuscular system.

REVIEW QUESTIONS

1. Chromium is a trace element important
   a. for cell growth and synthesis of carbohydrates.
   b. because it increases the effectiveness of insulin.
   c. because it assists in regulating osmotic pressure.
   d. in the formation of red blood cells.

2. Mr. J. is admitted with dehydration. His lab values are Na^+ 145 mEq/liter, K^+ 6 mEq/liter, Cl^- 95 mEq/liter, Mg^{++} 2.0 mEq/liter. Identify the electrolyte imbalance Mr. J. is experiencing.
   a. Hypernatremia.
   b. Hyperkalemia.
   c. Hypochloremia.
   d. Hypomagnesemia.

3. The drug of choice for treating hyperkalemia is
   a. sodium bicarbonate.
   b. deferoxamine (Desferal mesylate).
   c. pencillamine (Cuprimine).
   d. sodium polystyrene sulfonate (Kayexalate).

4. Inadequate ingestion of iron can result in
   a. heart failure.
   b. respiratory failure.
   c. inadequate oxygen supply to cells.
   d. decreased muscle mass.

5. Iodine can be found in
   a. citrus fruits.
   b. milk and eggs.
   c. wheat germ.
   d. red meat.

6. A zinc deficiency can cause
   a. thyroid enlargement.
   b. sensory impairment.
   c. stomatitis.
   d. lymphadenopathy.

7. Mrs. G. is being discharged on a potassium supplement along with a thiazide diuretic. Which of the following statements by Mrs. G. leads you to believe that she has understood the teaching you have done?

    a. "I will check my pulse regularly and contact my physician if there is a significant change."

    b. "I can take the potassium with vitamin C to increase its absorption."

    c. "I will take the medication on an empty stomach an hour before meals."

    d. "I can expect an increase in my appetite in about a week."

8. Symptoms of hypernatremia the nurse needs to observe for, when saline cathartics are administered, include

    a. bradycardia.

    b. diarrhea.

    c. hyperactive reflexes.

    d. headache and dizziness.

9. A person with hyperkalemia should be observed for

    a. muscle rigidity.

    b. hypertension.

    c. respiratory insufficiency.

    d. seizures.

10. The drug of choice for acute iron intoxication is

    a. sodium bicarbonate.

    b. succimer (Chemet).

    c. penicillamine (Cuprimine).

    d. deferoxamine (Desferal mesylate).

CRITICAL THINKING CASE STUDY

Mr. B. is seen in the emergency room for chest pain. He has not been feeling well for some time. He has been treated for hypertension for 5 years. His blood pressure is 170/90 and pulse is 110. Laboratory values are BUN 108 mg/dl, creatinine 10 mg/dl, sodium 142 mEq/liter, and potassium 7 mEq/liter.

1. Identify and prioritize your nursing actions.

The physician diagnoses Mr. B. with renal failure and orders sodium bicarbonate 45 mEq over 15 minutes and 5 ml of 10% calcium gluconate.

2. Identify what you will be assessing for.

Mr. B.'s potassium comes down to 5.9 mEq/liter. His physician orders Kayexalate in sorbitol via enema. Mr. B. asks you why the medication must be administered this way.

3. Describe how you will respond to Mr. B.'s inquiry.

VI

DRUGS USED TO TREAT INFECTIONS

33

General Characteristics of Antimicrobial Drugs

FILL IN THE BLANKS

Complete the following sentences.

1. Factors that predispose one to infection include

   a. _____

   b. _____

   c. _____

   d. _____

   e. _____

   f. _____

   g. _____

   h. _____

   i. _____

2. A hospital-acquired infection is also referred to as a _____ infection.

3. Antimicrobial drugs include

   _____, _____, and _____.

4. The term _____ refers to killing microorganisms.

5. The term _____ refers to inhibition of growth of microorganisms.

6. For most acute infections, the average duration of treatment with an antibiotic is _____ days.

7. If your client has renal insufficiency, the dose of the antibiotic may need to be _____. The drug dosage is based on the individual's _____ clearance.

8. Drugs that may cause nephrotoxicity and ototoxicity include _____.

9. Most oral anti-infectives should be given _____ before meals with _____ ounces of H_2O.

10. Adverse effects of antibiotics that the nurse should observe for include _____, _____, _____, and _____.

11. Common symptoms that can be seen with a superinfection are

    a. _____

    b. _____

    c. _____

    d. _____

    e. _____

REVIEW QUESTIONS

1. If your client has severe liver disease, the dose of antibiotic ordered may need to be
   a. increased.
   b. decreased.
   c. unchanged.
   d. withheld.

2. Persons in hospitals who are immunosuppressed are susceptible to this type of infection.
   a. Nosocomial infection.
   b. Communal infection.
   c. Sustained infection.
   d. Antimicrobial infection.

3. For most acute infections, the usual duration of treatment is
   a. 48–72 hours.
   b. 3–5 days.
   c. 7–10 days.
   d. 2–3 weeks.

4. Vaginal *Candida albicans* infection, commonly treated with miconazole (Monistat), is an example of a
   a. gram-positive bacterial infection.
   b. gram-negative bacterial infection.
   c. fungal infection.
   d. viral infection.

5. The following antimicrobial is contraindicated in children under the age of eight:
   a. Penicillin.
   b. Cephalosporins.
   c. Erythromycin.
   d. Tetracyclines.

6. The following impairs the body's defense mechanism and makes it more likely that an individual will develop an opportunistic infection:
   a. Therapy with thiazide diuretics.
   b. Weight loss.
   c. Dehydration.
   d. Chronic steroid drug therapy.

7. Objective signs of an infection include which of the following?
   a. Lethargy.
   b. Nausea.
   c. Leukocytosis.
   d. Hypertension.

8. Prophylactic antibiotics are used with dental procedures for persons with a history of
   a. diabetes mellitus.
   b. renal insufficiency.
   c. asthma.
   d. rheumatic heart disease.

9. Staphylococci normally found in the intestine are referred to as
   a. opportunistic microorganisms.
   b. indigenous flora.
   c. resistant microorganisms.
   d. nosocomial infections.

10. You should assess Mr. J., age 75, for nephrotoxicity and ototoxicity when administering which of the following antimicrobials?
    a. Cefazolin.
    b. Clindamycin.
    c. Gentamicin.
    d. Erythromycin.

34

Beta-Lactam Antibacterials: Penicillins, Cephalosporins, and Others

FILL IN THE BLANKS

Complete the following sentences.

1. Penicillins are the drugs of choice for treating

   a. _____

   b. _____

   c. _____

   d. _____

2. Penicillin is useful in _____,

   _____, or _____

   infections.

3. If an infection is caused by staphylococci that
   are resistant to penicillin G, the following drugs
   may be effective: _____,

   _____, _____,

   _____, and _____.

4. A broad spectrum, semisynthetic penicillin used
   for several types of gram-positive and gram-negative bacteria is _____.

5. Ampicillin is effective in treating the following
   infections: _____,

   _____, _____,

   and _____.

6. Unasyn is a combination of _____

   and _____.

7. Four penicillins used to treat *Pseudomonas* are

   _____, _____,

   _____, and _____.

8. Cephalosporins act against _____

   and _____ organisms.

9. There are _____, _____,

   _____, and _____

   generation cephalosporins.

10. Cephalosporins are commonly used for surgical
    prophylaxis and infections of the

    a. _____

    b. _____

    c. _____

    d. _____

    e. _____

    f. _____

11. A new carbapene used before causative organ-
    isms are identified is _____

    (_____).

CROSSWORD PUZZLE

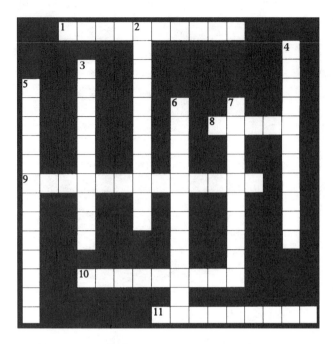

Across

1. A patient with an anaphylactic reaction to _____ may be sensitive to cephalosporins as well.

8. Cephalosporins may aggravate _____ impairment.

9. Third-generation cephalosporins can penetrate into _____ fluid and aid meningeal infections.

10. Preferred for intramuscular administration.

11. Contains amoxicillin and potassium clavulanate.

Down

2. The first third-generation cephalosporin approved for once daily dosage.

3. First-generation cephalosporins are often used to prevent infections after _____ surgery.

4. A penicillin that is effective against *Pseudomonas*.

5. These drugs decrease the effects of cephalosporins.

6. This drug is excreted in bile and its half-life is prolonged in hepatic failure.

7. The first oral cephalosporin, still extensively used.

REVIEW QUESTIONS

1. A penicillin used to treat staphylococcal infections that are resistant to penicillin G is
   a. bacampicillin (Spectrobid).
   b. amoxicillin (Amoxil).
   c. nafcillin (Unipen).
   d. carbenicillin (Geopen).

2. Your client weighs 132 lb and is to receive four doses of Unipen. The total daily dose is 50 mg/kg/day. How much will your client receive per dose?
   a. 500 mg.
   b. 750 mg.
   c. 2000 mg.
   d. 3000 mg.

3. After receiving penicillin for 5 days, Mrs. A. complains of soreness in her mouth, diarrhea, and vaginal itching, which may be signs of
   a. anaphylactic reactions to the drug.
   b. spread of her infection.
   c. ineffectiveness of drug therapy.
   d. superimposed infection.

4. When probenecid is administered with penicillin, the following results:
   a. Hypersensitivity is common.
   b. Glucosuria.
   c. Drug action is decreased.
   d. Drug action is increased.

5. A severe adverse reaction that someone might develop after the administration of a cephalosporin is
   a. hypertension.
   b. pseudomembranous colitis.
   c. diabetes mellitus.
   d. gingivitis.

6. Cefuroxime is used for surgical prophylaxis. When is the best time to administer the medication?
   a. 12 hours before surgery.
   b. 2 hours before surgery.
   c. 30–60 minutes before surgery.
   d. During surgery.

7. When administering large doses of cefamandole (Mandol) IV, the nurse needs to observe for

   a. tachycardia.

   b. jaundice.

   c. bleeding.

   d. hypertension.

8. Which of the following drugs, when administered with cephalosporins, will decrease their effects?

   a. Furosemide (Lasix).

   b. Probenecid (Benemid).

   c. Aminoglycosides.

   d. Tetracyclines.

9. Which of the following would be indicative of a cephalosporin allergy and should be reported to the physician?

   a. Nausea, vomiting, and diarrhea.

   b. Flushing, and swelling of the head and neck.

   c. Nasal congestion and itching.

   d. Skin rash, drug fever, and eosinophilia.

10. Which of the following instructions should be given to Mr. P., who is to be discharged on oral cephalosporins?

    a. "If you see blood, pus, or mucus in your stool, contact the doctor immediately."

    b. "Take the medication on an empty stomach to increase its absorption."

    c. "Do not use antacids while you are taking this medication."

    d. "If your urinary output decreases, cut the dose of the medication in half."

CRITICAL THINKING CASE STUDY

Mr. B., a type I diabetic, is admitted to the hospital with severe dehydration. He has recently returned from a trip and has had diarrhea since he returned home. His stool culture reveals *Shigella,* and he is started on ampicillin and sulbactam (Unasyn) IV.

1. Explain why this drug was chosen for Mr. B.

2. Explain the rationale for the route of administration.

The following morning, you enter Mr. B.'s room and find that Mr. B. has a dull red rash on his face and chest.

3. Identify and prioritize your nursing activities.

35

Aminoglycosides and Fluoroquinolones

FILL IN THE BLANKS

Complete the following sentences.

1. Aminoglycosides are used to treat infections caused by _____ microorganisms.

2. Quinolones are commonly used to treat _____ infections.

3. Aminoglycosides are used intravenously to treat _____ and _____ infections.

4. Streptomycin is used for tuberculosis that is _____.

5. Aminoglycosides are also used orally to suppress _____, which produce _____.

6. Neomycin is recommended for _____ or _____ administration only. Neomycin is used to treat infections of the _____, _____, and _____.

7. Before administering aminoglycosides, the nurse should

    a. _____

    b. _____

    c. analyze medications and assess other drugs that may be _____

    d. _____

8. While your client is receiving aminoglycosides, monitor _____ and _____, and force fluids to _____ daily.

9. Fluoroquinolones are used to treat infections caused by _____ organisms.

10. Fluoroquinolones are contraindicated in

    a. _____

    b. _____

    c. _____

11. Peak levels should be obtained _____ minutes after a dose. Both peak and _____ levels are necessary to establish a therapeutic serum level. Trough levels are taken 10–15 minutes before the next dose. For gentamicin and tobramycin, peak levels above _____ µg/ml and trough levels above _____ µg/ml have been associated with nephrotoxicity.

12. When administering aminoglycosides, avoid concurrent administration with _____.

REVIEW QUESTIONS

1. Aminoglycosides are used orally to treat
    a. gram-positive bacteria.
    b. gram-negative bacteria.
    c. fungal infections.
    d. viral infections.

2. The physician orders gentamicin for a child weighing 88 lb. If the dose range is 6–7.5 mg/kg/day, and the child is to receive the medication t.i.d., how many milligrams should the child receive per dose?

    a. 20 mg.

    b. 40 mg.

    c. 60 mg.

    d. 80 mg.

3. Which of the following drugs should be avoided when a person is receiving aminoglycosides?

    a. Furosemide (Lasix).

    b. Prednisone.

    c. Aspirin.

    d. Propranolol (Inderal).

4. Aminoglycosides can be nephrotoxic. The most effective way of preventing compromised renal function in Mr. T. is to

    a. maintain his pulse above 60.

    b. keep him well hydrated.

    c. provide daily exercise to ensure adequate blood flow to the kidneys.

    d. avoid concurrent administration of aminoglycosides with antacids.

5. An aminoglycoside that is used in hepatic coma to decrease intestinal bacteria is

    a. paromomycin sulfate (Humatin).

    b. netilmicin (Netromycin).

    c. streptomycin.

    d. tobramycin (Nebcin).

6. This drug is commonly used with gentamicin (Garamycin) to treat *Pseudomonas* infections.

    a. Ticarcillin (Ticar).

    b. Moxalactam (Moxam).

    c. Ceftriaxone (Rocephin).

    d. Cephradine (Anspor).

7. Trough serum drug levels for gentamicin should be drawn

    a. 15 minutes before the next dose.

    b. 30 minutes before the next dose.

    c. 2 hours before the next dose.

    d. 1 hour before the next dose.

8. Which of the following lab studies is indicative of nephrotoxicity?

    a. Elevated WBC.

    b. Increased serum potassium.

    c. Increased serum creatinine.

    d. Elevated serum sodium.

9. When administering aminoglycosides, avoid concurrent administration of the following agents because they may produce paralysis of respiratory muscles:

    a. Penicillin.

    b. Beta-blockers.

    c. Calcium channel blockers.

    d. Quinidine.

10. Mr. J. has a peak gentamicin level of 14 µg/ml. This level is

    a. within the therapeutic range.

    b. lower than the therapeutic range.

    c. slightly above the therapeutic range.

    d. associated with nephrotoxicity.

CRITICAL THINKING CASE STUDY

Mrs. J. is being treated with tobramycin (Nebcin) for a *Pseudomonas* infection.

1. Identify the assessments that will be done before and during treatment with this drug.

Mrs. J.'s urinary output begins to drop.

2. Identify your nursing actions.

You speak to the physician on call about Mrs. J.'s decreased urinary output. He orders Lasix 80 mg IV push.

3. Discuss what you will do next.

36

Tetracyclines, Sulfonamides and Urinary Agents

FILL IN THE BLANKS

Complete the following sentences.

1. Tetracyclines are effective against _____ and _____ organisms as well as _____, _____, some _____, _____, and others.

2. The older tetracyclines are excreted mainly in _____; the newer ones are mainly excreted in _____.

3. Tetracyclines are the first drug of choice for
   a. _____
   b. _____
   c. _____
   d. _____
   e. _____
   f. _____
   g. _____

4. _____ may be used in the management of _____ inappropriate ADH secretion.

5. If tetracyclines are administered to children, they can cause _____ and may _____.

6. Sulfonamides should be used with caution in the presence of _____ or _____ impairment or _____.

7. During sulfonamide therapy, fluids should be forced to prevent _____.

8. Oral tetracycline preparations should be administered _____.

9. Tetracyclines should not be administered with _____.

10. When taking tetracycline, you should avoid exposure to _____ because it may cause _____ or _____.

11. Sulfonamides are _____ not bactericidal.

12. Sulfonamides are often used in the treatment of _____ infections.

13. Two drugs that increase the effects of tetracycline include _____ and _____.

14. Give nitrofurantoin _____ meals to prevent _____, _____, and _____.

15. Persons taking tetracycline should report the following symptoms of a superinfection to the physician: _____, _____, _____, _____, _____, or itching in the _____ area.

16. Do not take _____ products with tetracycline because they will produce non-absorbable compounds.

17. Persons taking medications for a urinary tract infection should drink _____.

CROSSWORD PUZZLE

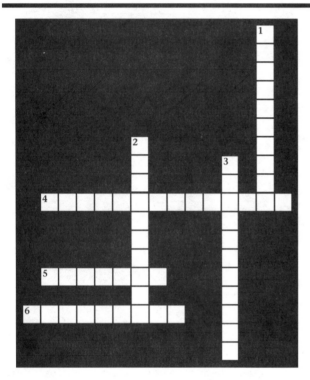

Across

4. The tetracycline most likely to cause photosensitivity.
5. Used for otitis media in children.
6. Topical application is painless.

Down

1. Available for ocular infections.
2. Used for ulcerative colitis.
3. Prevents bacterial colonization of wounds.

REVIEW QUESTIONS

1. You know your health teaching has been effective if your client, who is taking doxycycline (Vibramycin), states she should
   a. take the drug with food.
   b. contact the physician if she develops acne.
   c. only take it if she is going to be inside all day.
   d. take vitamin supplements with the medication.

2. If tetracycline is administered to children under 8, it can cause
   a. muscle weakness.
   b. renal insufficiency.
   c. gastrointestinal bleeding.
   d. permanent yellow-gray discoloration of the teeth.

3. Sulfisoxazole (Gantrisin) is prescribed for Mrs. P. What information should you give to Mrs. P.?
   a. "Since depression of bone can occur, take this drug for no more than 22 weeks."
   b. "Headache and dizziness are expected the first few days."
   c. "Be careful of over the counter medications because aspirin can increase toxicity of sulfonamides."
   d. "You must drink eight glasses of water daily when you take this drug."

4. Which of the following sulfonamides is used in the management of Crohn's disease?
   a. Sulfadiazine (Microsulfon).
   b. Sulfisoxazole (Gantrisin).
   c. Sulfamethoxazole-trimethoprim (Septra).
   d. Sulfasalazine (Azulfidine).

5. The only tetracycline that can be given safely to an individual who has renal impairment is
   a. minocycline (Minocin).
   b. oxytetracycline (Terramycin).
   c. methacycline (Rondomycin).
   d. doxycycline (Vibramycin).

6. Mrs. J., who is 6 months pregnant, comes to the doctor asking for a prescription for tetracycline to treat her acne. Your response should be

   a. "Tetracycline, if taken during pregnancy, will be deposited in the bones and teeth of the fetus."

   b. "Tetracycline can cause renal failure if taken during pregnancy."

   c. "The effect of tetracycline is decreased during pregnancy."

   d. "Taking tetracycline during pregnancy can cause premature labor."

7. When caring for a client taking tetracycline, you should assess him or her for symptoms of a superinfection, which include

   a. headache.

   b. sore mouth.

   c. decreased urinary output.

   d. blurred vision.

8. Which drug, if administered with a sulfonamide, will decrease its actions?

   a. Aspirin.

   b. Propranolol (Inderal).

   c. Furosemide (Lasix).

   d. Maalox.

9. When administering tetracycline, the nurse should observe Mr. C. for adverse effects of the medication, which include

   a. confusion.

   b. adrenal insufficiency.

   c. hepatotoxicity.

   d. elevated blood sugars.

10. Tetracycline is the drug of choice for treating

   a. typhus and cholera.

   b. respiratory tract infections.

   c. infections of the soft tissue.

   d. septicemia.

CRITICAL THINKING CASE STUDY

M.J., a 16-year-old high school student, comes to the dermatologist to be treated for acne. She is given a prescription for tetracycline.

1. Identify the assessments that will be done before she starts the medication.

2. Discuss the instructions you will give M.J. before she starts the medication.

M.J. returns to the office in 4 weeks and states that the medication has been ineffective.

3. Identify the information you will elicit from M.J. to help make your assessment.

After additional instructions, M.J. decides to continue the medication. She returns to the office 4 weeks later complaining of a sore throat.

4. Identify your nursing actions.

37

Macrolides and Miscellaneous Antibacterials

FILL IN THE BLANKS

Complete the following sentences.

1. Erythromycin and clindamycin are
   _____ rather than bactericidal
   except in _____ doses.

2. Clinical indications for using erythromycin
   include
   a. _____
   b. _____
   c. _____
   d. _____
   e. _____
   f. _____
   g. _____
   h. _____

3. Azithromycin (_____) and clar-
   ithromycin (_____) are indicated for treating _____.

4. Chloramphenicol (_____) is
   the drug of choice for _____.

5. Clindamycin (_____) is useful
   as a penicillin substitute in persons who have
   _____, _____,
   or _____ infections.

6. _____ (_____)
   is used to treat methicillin-resistant *Staphylococ-
   cus aureus* infection.

7. Initial treatment for *C. difficile* colitis is metronidazole (_____).

8. Erythromycin should be administered on
   _____ stomach.

9. Common side effects of macrolides are
   _____, _____,
   and _____.

10. Symptoms of hepatotoxicity include
    _____, _____,
    _____, _____,
    _____, and _____.

TRUE OR FALSE

1. _____ Erythromycin is used as a substitute for
   penicillin.

2. _____ In renal failure, the dosage of erythromycin needs to be reduced.

3. _____ If an aminoglycoside is administered with
   erythromycin, it will decrease the effect of
   the erythromycin.

4. _____ Red man syndrome is caused by rapid
   infusion of vancomycin and results in
   hypotension and skin flushing.

5. _____ Diarrhea may occur with topical clindamycin for treatment of acne.

REVIEW QUESTIONS

1. The nurse should observe for this common adverse effect related to the administration of erythromycin:

   a. vomiting.

   b. elevated blood sugar.

   c. elevated uric acid levels.

   d. decreased WBC.

2. Which of the following medications will increase the effect of erythromycin when administered with it?

   a. Streptomycin.

   b. Tetracycline.

   c. Aztreonam (Azactam).

   d. Ceftriaxone (Rocephin).

3. Erythromycin is used as a substitute treatment for persons allergic to penicillin to treat

   a. glomerulonephritis.

   b. peritonitis.

   c. fungal infections.

   d. gonorrhea and syphilis.

4. A nursing measure that will help minimize the adverse effects associated with the administration of vancomycin is

   a. observe for convulsions, dizziness, and headaches.

   b. assess intake and output and serum creatinine levels.

   c. administer the medication over 4 hours.

   d. assess breath sounds during administration of the medication.

5. Phlebitis associated with the administration of IV erythromycin may be decreased by

   a. decreasing the amount of solution administered with the drug.

   b. applying warm compresses to the site during the infusion.

   c. administering the IV medication slowly.

   d. infusing the medication in 1000 cc of IV fluid over 8 hours.

6. The physician's order reads: Administer clindamycin (Cleocin) 600 mg in 100 cc over 20 minutes. Using macro drip tubing (10 gtt = 1 cc), how fast will you run the IV?

   a. 20 gtt/minute.

   b. 30 gtt/minute.

   c. 40 gtt/minute.

   d. 50 gtt/minute.

7. Symptoms of pseudomembranous colitis that can result because of administration of clindamycin (Cleocin) include

   a. ascites and peripheral edema.

   b. hypertension and constipation.

   c. diarrhea, fever, and blood in stools.

   d. nausea, vomiting, and abdominal cramps.

8. M.J., who weighs 66 lb, is to receive clindamycin palmitate hydrochloride (Cleocin) in three divided doses. The maximum dose for a child her size is 25 mg/kg/day. If the pediatric Cleocin medication comes at 75 mg/ml, how many milliliters will M.J. receive per dose?

   a. 1.6 ml.

   b. 2.8 ml.

   c. 3.3 ml.

   d. 4.5 ml.

9. J.R., age 13, is being treated with clindamycin (Cleocin) for acne. Which of the following statements leads you to believe that he has understood the teaching you have done?

   a. "I can only take this drug for 2 weeks because it causes depression of bone growth."

   b. "Headache and dizziness are expected the first few days I take this medication."

   c. "I will report severe vomiting, diarrhea, or a rash to my physician."

   d. "I will drink eight glasses of water daily while I am taking this medication."

10. A serum level of vancomycin is drawn, and it is 15 mcg/ml. This is

   a. below the therapeutic range.

   b. within the therapeutic range.

   c. slightly above the therapeutic range.

   d. within a toxic range.

CRITICAL THINKING CASE STUDY

Mr. R., a 40-year-old attorney, has been experiencing chills, fever, and lethargy for 2 days. He is seen by his physician in the office, diagnosed with pneumonia, and started on erythromycin.

1. Identify the initial assessments the physician would have done to establish this diagnosis.

2. Identify the instructions that you will give Mr. R. before he returns home.

Mrs. R. calls you the next day to tell you that her husband has been vomiting on and off since he started on the medication.

3. Specify what your instruction to Mrs. R. will be.

Mr. R. is admitted to the hospital and started on erythromycin IV. He continues to vomit.

4. Identify what you will do.

38

Drugs for Tuberculosis and Mycobacterium Avium Complex (MAC) Disease

8. The following reactions to antitubercular drugs should be reported to the physician:

   a. _____

   b. _____

   c. _____

   d. _____

   e. _____

   f. _____

FILL IN THE BLANKS

Complete the following sentences.

1. Today, the recommended length of initial treatment for TB is _____ months.

2. The primary drugs used for initial treatment are _____, _____, _____, and _____.

3. Secondary drugs are used when _____.

4. An indication for prophylactic use of INH would be a positive _____.

5. For persons exposed to someone with MDR-TB, _____ and _____ may be given.

6. The dosage of ethambutol is calculated according to _____.

7. Rifampin should be administered _____ or _____ a meal.

MATCHING EXERCISE

Match each drug with the associated effects or information.

1. _____ INH.

2. _____ Rifampin.

3. _____ Pyrazinamide.

4. _____ Ethambutol.

5. _____ Rifamate.

6. _____ Rifabutin.

A. Causes a reddish-orange discoloration of body fluids.

B. Can affect red–green visual discrimination.

C. Accelerates the metabolism of several drugs.

D. A combination product.

E. Can cause hepatotoxicity and peripheral neuropathy.

F. Causes hyperuricemia.

IDENTIFY THE TREATMENT

Place an A in the table for drugs that are used alone to treat exposures to active TB and a C in the table for drugs that are used in combination. Use an asterisk to indicate that use of either drug is appropriate and a checkmark to indicate "may also be used."

	INH	Rifampin	Etham-butol	Pyrazin-amide	Ofloxacin	Strepto-mycin	Amikacin	Cipro-floxacin
1. Exposed to TB with a negative chest x-ray								
2. Exposed to TB that is INH resistant								
3. Exposed to MDR TB								
4. Initial diagnosis of active TB								
5. Active MDR TB								
6. Active TB during pregnancy								

REVIEW QUESTIONS

1. What findings would lead you to believe that your client may be experiencing hepatic toxicity from isoniazid (INH)?

   a. Diarrhea.

   b. Numbness and tingling.

   c. Visual disturbances.

   d. Dark urine.

2. Which of the following drugs should be taken on an empty stomach to prevent delayed absorption?

   a. Rifampin (Rifadin).

   b. Para-amino salicylic acid (PAS).

   c. INH (Laniazid).

   d. Streptomycin.

3. Early symptoms of a hypersensitivity reaction to antitubercular drugs are likely to occur between

   a. 48 and 72 hours after initiation of drug therapy.

   b. the third and eighth weeks of drug therapy.

   c. a week and 10 days after initiation of drug therapy.

   d. the second and third month of drug therapy.

4. Which of the following statements by your client, who has active TB, leads you to believe that she has a good understanding of how she is to take the medication?

   a. "I will take the medication until the symptoms subside."

   b. "I may have to take as many as four medications for 4 months."

   c. "I will take the medication for 6 months and then I am finished."

   d. "I will take a combination of medications for 9 months to 2 years."

5. Which of the following statements is true regarding tuberculosis?

   a. Symptoms of TB occur within 2 weeks of exposure.

   b. TB affects only the lungs.

   c. TB can be controlled by chemotherapy.

   d. TB can be cured with radiation therapy.

6. Therapeutic effects of antitubercular drug therapy include

   a. increased cough, sputum, and night sweats.

   b. decreased appetite and weight.

   c. positive cultures.

   d. no changes in chest x-ray.

7. When taking INH (Laniazid), which of the following things should Mr. C. be instructed to avoid?

    a. Alcohol.

    b. Caffeine.

    c. Dairy products.

    d. Citrus fruits.

8. You are doing the discharge teaching of a person newly diagnosed with TB. You need to tell him that the usual length of time that persons must take isoniazid (INH) is

    a. 10 days.

    b. 3 months.

    c. 6 months.

    d. 1 year.

9. Mr. J. weighs 143 lb and the recommended daily dose of ethambutol (Myambutol) is 15 mg/kg/day. How many milligrams should he receive daily?

    a. 500 mg.

    b. 650 mg.

    c. 975 mg.

    d. 1250 mg.

10. Which of the following statements by Mrs. G. leads you to believe that she had understood the teaching you have done regarding rifampin (Rifadin)?

    a. "Dizziness, drowsiness, and decreased urinary output are common with this drug, but they will subside over time."

    b. "Constipation will be a problem so I will increase the fiber in my diet."

    c. "Initially, I may experience blurred vision and inability to distinguish colors, but it will improve in a few weeks."

    d. "This medication may cause my bodily secretions to turn red."

CRITICAL THINKING CASE STUDY

Miss G., a 25-year-old public health nurse, has a positive tuberculin test but a negative chest x-ray. She is started on INH.

1. Identify what your instruction will be for Miss G.

Miss G. calls your office 2 months after starting the medication and states that she has stopped menstruating and that her skin has a yellow cast.

2. Identify your response.

39

Antiviral Drugs

13. _____ Repeated courses of acyclovir (Zovirax) therapy may result in severe anemia and granulocytopenia.

14. _____ Seizures are associated with high plasma levels of amantadine (Symmetrel).

15. _____ Nevirapine is indicated for clients with advanced HIV infections whose condition is worsening.

MATCHING EXERCISE

Terms and Concepts

Match each drug with the adverse effects associated with it.

1. _____ Acyclovir (Zovirax).

2. _____ Amantadine (Symmetrel).

3. _____ Ganciclovir (Cytovene).

4. _____ Ribavirin (Vibrazole).

5. _____ Idoxuridine (Herplex).

A. Insomnia, ataxia, and slurred speech.

B. Respiratory distress.

C. Pain, itching, and inflammation of eyelids.

D. Anemia, neutropenia, and thrombocytopenia.

E. Lethargy, confusion, and seizures.

TRUE OR FALSE

1. _____ Viruses can live for hours outside of a living organism.

2. _____ Acyclovir (Zovirax) inactivates the herpes virus and prevents the recurrence of the disease.

3. _____ Amantadine (Symmetrel) may be useful in the treatment of influenza A infections.

4. _____ Ganciclovir (Cytovene) is effective in curing CMV retinitis.

5. _____ Ribavirin (Virazole) is administered by inhalation for the treatment of RSV infection.

6. _____ Zidovudine (AZT) was the first anti-HIV drug developed.

7. _____ Stavudine may be used with didanosine to prevent peripheral neuropathy.

8. _____ Ophthalmic antiviral preparations such as trifluridine can cause ocular toxicity.

9. _____ Persons who have visible herpes lesions will not spread the disease if they apply acyclovir before having sexual intercourse.

10. _____ There are many vaccines available that will prevent viral diseases including poliomyelitis, mumps, yellow fever, and rabies.

11. _____ Zidovudine (AZT), when used for persons with AIDS, prevents the occurrence of opportunistic infections.

12. _____ Viral infections can occur without any signs and symptoms of illness.

REVIEW QUESTIONS

1. Adverse effects of acyclovir (Zovirax) that the nurse needs to assess for include

   a. increased serum creatinine.

   b. thrombocytopenia.

   c. respiratory distress.

   d. psychosis.

2. An expected outcome after the administration of acyclovir (Zovirax) for genital herpes is

   a. decreased fever.

   b. decreased pain.

   c. prevention of recurrence.

   d. smaller size of lesion during next exacerbation.

3. Live attenuated viral vaccines should not be administered to persons who are receiving

   a. oral hypoglycemic agents.

   b. antineoplastic agents.

   c. intravenous antibiotics.

   d. pulmonary bronchodilators.

4. Which of the following statements by Mr. J. leads you to believe that he understands how to use trifluridine (Viroptic)?

   a. "After I take this medication, I may notice burning, stinging, or eyelid edema."

   b. "Each time after I administer the medication, I will apply cold compresses to my eyes."

   c. "I should use this drug for no longer than 10 days because it can cause ocular toxicity."

   d. "I will use the medication once a day before I go to bed."

5. Which of the following statements by your client with AIDS leads you to believe that he needs additional teaching?

   a. "Zidovudine (AZT) may need to be stopped temporarily if bone marrow depression occurs."

   b. "Zidovudine (AZT) therapy may result in the development of anemia."

   c. "Zidovudine (AZT) slows the progression of the disease but does not cure it."

   d. "Zidovudine (AZT) prevents the transmission of the virus through sexual contact."

6. Ribavirin (Virazole) for treatment of respiratory syncytial viral infections is administered via

   a. the rectum.

   b. an intravenous route.

   c. subcutaneous injection.

   d. inhalation.

7. You are to administer acyclovir (Zovirax) intravenously. The recommended dose is 5 mg/kg q8h. Your client weighs 110 lb. How much medication will you administer per day?

   a. 250 mg.

   b. 500 mg.

   c. 750 mg.

   d. 1000 mg.

8. For which of the following disorders in Mr. G.'s history would you contact the doctor before administering amantadine (Symmetrel)?

   a. Allergies to pollen and dog dander.

   b. Epilepsy.

   c. Diabetes mellitus.

   d. Chronic lung disease.

9. Which of the following medications, if administered concurrently with zidovudine (AZT), will increase its effects?

   a. Acetaminophen (Tylenol).

   b. Atropine.

   c. Amphotericin B.

   d. Propranolol (Inderal).

10. Which of the following medications, if administered with amantadine (Symmetrel), will cause blurred vision, dry mouth, and urine retention?

   a. Atropine.

   b. Furosemide (Lasix).

   c. Prednisone.

   d. Sodium bicarbonate.

CRITICAL THINKING CASE STUDY

J.J., a 32-year-old male, has recently been diagnosed with HIV infection and is started on zidovudine (AZT).

1. Discuss the instructions that you will give him.

2. Identify three nursing diagnoses that would be appropriate for J.J.

J.J.'s disease progresses rapidly. Within 3 years, he develops AIDS and has contracted several opportunistic infections. He is presently being seen for cytomegalovirus retinitis, for which the doctor orders ganciclovir (Cytovene).

3. Discuss the instructions that you will give him.

J.J. calls you because he has noticed some bleeding. He is crying on the phone and states, "I don't want to die."

4. Discuss how you will respond to J.J.

40

Antifungal Drugs

MATCHING EXERCISE

Terms and Concepts

Match the concept with the term for it.

1. _____ Tinea pedis.

2. _____ A highly contagious fungal infection spread by sharing towels and hairbrushes.

3. _____ Thrush.

4. _____ This can occur as a result of the administration of total parenteral nutrition.

5. _____ Found in soil and organic debris.

6. _____ Causes a respiratory infection that resembles pneumonia or tuberculosis.

7. _____ Used to treat fungal infections of the eye.

8. _____ Drug used to treat athlete's foot.

9. _____ Can cause hypokalemia and anemia.

10. _____ Drug administered intravenously to treat systemic mycoses.

11. _____ Adverse effects of this drug include nausea, vomiting, pruritus, and abdominal pain.

12. _____ Serious adverse effects resulting from the administration of this drug include mental confusion and blood dyscrasias.

13. _____ The length of time antifungal drugs are administered.

14. _____ Signs and symptoms of histoplasmosis, coccidioidomycosis, and blastomycosis.

15. _____ A drug used for the treatment of vaginal candidiasis.

16. _____ Fungi that cause superficial skin infections.

17. _____ Can occur following inhalation of airborne spores from air conditioning units.

18. _____ This drug will increase the effects of fluconazole.

A. Athlete's foot.

B. Amphotericin B (Fungizone).

C. Blastomycosis.

D. Miconazole (Monistat).

E. Haloprogin (Halotex).

F. Oral candidiasis.

G. Tinea capitis.

H. Natamycin (Natacyn).

I. Fungus causing histoplasmosis.

J. Systemic candidiasis.

K. Griseofulvin (Fulvicin).

L. 7–10 days.

M. 2–6 weeks.

N. Cough, fever, malaise.

O. Ketoconazole.

P. Vaginal discharge, burning, itching.

Q. Clotrimazole (Lotrimin).

R. Aspergillosis.

S. Dermatophytes.

T. Hydrochlorothiazide.

FILL IN THE BLANKS

Complete the following sentences.

1. Mechanisms of contracting a fungal infection include _____, _____, and _____.

2. Drugs used for superficial fungal infections of the skin are usually administered _____.

3. Exposure to pigeon, chicken, or bat excreta can result in _____.

4. Corticosteroid use can lead to a _____ infection.

5. _____ is a potent intravenous antifungal drug used for serious systemic infections.

REVIEW QUESTIONS

1. The drug most commonly used to treat tinea pedis is
   a. acrisorcin (Akrinol).
   b. tolnaftate (Tinactin).
   c. griseofulvin (Fulvicin).
   d. nystatin (Mycostatin).

2. Your client weighs 88 lb and is to receive amphotericin B (Fungizone) 0.50 mg/kg daily. If she receives two doses daily, how much medication will she receive per dose?
   a. 10 mg.
   b. 20 mg.
   c. 100 mg.
   d. 200 mg.

3. Which of the following medications, if administered concurrently with amphotericin B, may increase nephrotoxicity?
   a. Aminoglycosides.
   b. Antipyretics.
   c. Beta-adrenergic blockers.
   d. Potassium-sparing diuretics.

4. Your client is receiving intravenous amphotericin B (Fungizone). He should be observed for
   a. tachycardia.
   b. an elevated creatinine level.
   c. a low serum sodium level.
   d. severe diarrhea.

5. Which of the following statements leads you to believe that your client has understood the teaching you have done regarding ketoconazole (Nizoral)?
   a. "I should take this medication with milk or an antacid to prevent gastrointestinal upset."
   b. "I know that as a result of taking this medication, I could develop nausea, vomiting, and abdominal pain."
   c. "I know that I will need to take this medication for a week to 10 days, but no longer."
   d. "I know that as a result of taking this medication, I could develop a resistance to this medication."

6. Which of the following medications, if administered concurrently with griseofulvin (Fulvicin), will decrease its effect?
   a. Cephalothin (Keflin).
   b. Furosemide (Lasix).
   c. Prednisone.
   d. Phenobarbital.

7. Which of the following is a drug of choice for treating histoplasmosis?
   a. Acrisorcin (Akrinol).
   b. Flucytosine (Ancobon).
   c. Natamycin (Natacyn).
   d. Ketoconazole (Nizoral).

8. Which of the following instructions will you give your client regarding administration of acrisorcin (Akrinol)?
   a. Apply the ointment to the lesions for 3 months.
   b. Apply the medication to the skin lesions twice a day for 6 weeks.
   c. Place the solution in a sitz bath and soak in it twice daily.
   d. Fill the applicator with the medication and apply the cream q4h and place sterile pads on the lesions after each treatment.

9. Which of the following statements by M.S. leads you to believe that she has understood the teaching you have done regarding the use of natamycin (Natacyn) for a fungal infection of her eye?
   a. "I will apply one drop to each eye q 1–2 hours for 3 days, then every 3–4 hours for 3 weeks."
   b. "I will take the medication orally, on an empty stomach, twice a day for 2 weeks."
   c. "After each application of the medication, I will apply cool compresses to my eyes."
   d. "I will rinse my eyes with the solution four times a day for 1 month."

10. Which of the following instructions should you give your client who is being treated with econazole (Spectazole) for ringworm?

a. Wash your head four times every day for 2 weeks.

b. Do not share towels with any other member of the family.

c. Do not eat meat while using this medication.

d. Comb the medication into your hair, then apply gauze over your head to keep from spreading it to the others.

CRITICAL THINKING CASE STUDY

M., a 32-year-old model, comes to the physician's office with a fungal infection of her fingernails caused by application of ceramic fingernails. The physician orders griseofulvin (Fulvicin). M. is leaving for a job in Hawaii and asks for a 4-week supply of the medication.

1. Discuss with M. why her plans concern you.

2. Identify the instructions that you will give M., including the adverse effects of griseofulvin (Fulvicin).

3. Identify three nursing diagnoses for M.

M. returns after her trip to Hawaii complaining of headache, dizziness, and fatigue.

4. Identify what you will do.

41

Antiparasitics

TRUE OR FALSE

1. _____ *Entamoeba histolytica* can live outside of the body for long periods.

2. _____ Amebiasis can result in abscesses of the lungs and brain.

3. _____ Malaria is a common cause of mortality and morbidity worldwide.

4. _____ Giardiasis is transmitted by the ingestion of improperly cooked beef, pork, or fish.

5. _____ Roundworms, caused by *Ascaris lumbricoides,* are the most common parasitic worm infections in the USA.

6. _____ Scabies and pediculosis can be transmitted by direct contact with the personal effects of an infected person.

7. _____ Parasitic worms can enter the bloodstream and migrate to other body tissues.

8. _____ Metronidazole stains feces a bright red color that can be mistaken for blood.

9. _____ Lindane (Kwell), used for the treatment of scabies, is absorbed through the skin and can produce CNS toxicity.

10. _____ Pyrimethamine (Daraprim) is used to treat malaria attacks.

11. _____ Visible skin lesions associated with scabies are commonly found between the fingers.

12. _____ Topical antitrichomonal agents can cause rash and inflammation.

13. _____ When a trichomonas infection is diagnosed, it is common practice to treat the sexual partner as well as the individual with the confirmed diagnosis.

14. _____ Quinine can also be used for treatment of nocturnal leg cramps.

15. _____ A person being treated for dwarf tapeworms with niclosamide (Niclocide) is not considered cured until he or she has negative stools for 3 months.

16. _____ Toxoplasmosis may be caused by contact with feces from infected cats.

REVIEW QUESTIONS

1. Mr. C. is being treated for amebiasis. The nurse should instruct him that the following adverse reactions are commonly experienced with amebicides:

   a. Tachycardia and hypotension.

   b. Oliguria and weight gain.

   c. Nausea, vomiting, and diarrhea.

   d. Dizziness and paresthesias.

2. Persons using iodoquinol (Yodoxin) should be instructed to report which of the following signs/symptoms to their physician?

   a. Fatigue.

   b. Decreased sensation in hands or feet.

   c. Headache and blurred vision.

   d. Anorexia.

3. Which of the following instructions should you give to Miss G., who is starting on a douche for trichomoniasis?

   a. Administer the douche daily for 1 month.

   b. Administer the douche three times a day for 1 week.

   c. Avoid sexual intercourse during treatment so that you can be sure you are free of infection.

   d. Wear gloves when administering the douche and keep it away from your perineal area.

4. P.G. is sent home with a note from school stating that she has pediculosis (head lice). Which of the following instructions should you give P.G.'s mother about the use of permethrin (Nix)?

   a. Apply to P.G.'s head three times a day for 2 weeks.

   b. Bathe P.G., apply Nix to all her body surfaces, leave it on for 24 hours, and bathe her again.

   c. Apply it to her scalp and hair; leave it on for 10 min, then rinse off with water.

   d. Have P.G. take a warm shower in the morning and apply Nix all over her body; repeat the procedure that evening.

5. Which of the following statements by a client being treated for pinworms leads you to believe that she has understood the teaching you have done regarding mebendazole (Vermox)?

   a. "I will need to have three negative stool cultures before I will be considered free of the pinworms."

   b. "I may continue to expel worms for 3 days after therapy is completed."

   c. "I will not drink alcohol when I am using this medication."

   d. "I will eat foods high in roughage to assist with passage of the worms."

6. Which of the following drugs, if taken with chloroquine phosphate (Aralen), will decrease its effects?

   a. Vitamin C (ascorbic acid).

   b. Vitamin E (Aquasol E).

   c. Furosemide (Lasix).

   d. Cephradine (Velosef).

7. Mr. B. is being treated for rheumatoid arthritis with hydroxychloroquine sulfate (Plaquenil). This drug should be used cautiously with which of the following disorders?

   a. Hypertension.

   b. Diabetes mellitus.

   c. Hepatic disease.

   d. Renal insufficiency.

8. Your client is diagnosed with trichomoniasis and started on metronidazole (Flagyl). Which of the following instructions should you give her?

   a. "Change your bed linens daily until the infection is gone."

   b. "Your partner should also be treated to prevent the possibility of reinfection."

   c. "You should refrain from sexual intercourse for 2 months."

   d. "You may gain 2–5 lb while on this medication, but you will lose the weight as soon as the medication is discontinued."

9. Mr. B. is receiving aerosol pentamidine (Nebu-Pent) for prophylaxis for *Pneumocystis carinii* pneumonia (PCP). He should be observed for adverse reactions to this medication, which include

   a. hypertension, tachycardia, and diarrhea.

   b. headache, tinnitus, and blurred vision.

   c. chest pain, dyspnea, and dizziness.

   d. weakness, constipation, and paresthesia.

10. Your client is taking metronidazole (Flagyl) for trichomoniasis. Which of the following statements leads you to believe that she has understood the teaching you have done?

   a. "I will limit my intake of caffeine while I am taking this medication."

   b. "I will eat a diet low in sodium while taking this medication."

   c. "I will increase my daily intake of potassium while taking this medication."

   d. "I will not drink any alcohol while taking this medication."

VII

DRUGS AFFECTING THE IMMUNE SYSTEM

42

Physiology of the Immune System

MATCHING EXERCISE

Terms and Concepts

Match the concept with the term for it.

1. _____ A generalized reaction to cellular injury from any cause.

2. _____ Stimulates production of antibodies that destroy foreign invaders.

3. _____ Detects and eliminates foreign substances that may cause tissue injury.

4. _____ Develops during gestation or after birth; may be active or passive.

5. _____ Occurs when antibodies are formed by the immune system of another person or animal and transferred to the host.

6. _____ Foreign substances that initiate immune responses.

7. _____ WBCs found throughout the body in lymphoid tissues.

8. _____ The first WBCs that start phagocytosis.

9. _____ WBCs that arrive later, ingest larger amounts of antigen, and have a longer life span than the first WBCs that respond.

10. _____ The primary regulator of the immune response.

11. _____ Originate in stem cells in bone marrow.

12. _____ Protein growth factors secreted by WBCs that stimulate leukocyte replication and function.

13. _____ Interfere with the ability of viruses to replicate in infected cells.

14. _____ Stimulate growth and differentiation of cells.

15. _____ A factor that affects immunologic response.

A. Immune response.

B. Passive immunity.

C. Antigens.

D. Inflammation.

E. Immune cells.

F. T lymphocytes.

G. Interferons.

H. Immune system.

I. Cytokines.

J. Acquired immunity.

K. Interleukins.

L. Monocytes.

M. Age.

N. B lymphocytes.

O. Neutrophils.

REVIEW QUESTIONS

1. Active immunity
   a. occurs when antibodies are formed by the immune system of another person and transferred to the host.
   b. develops within 6 months after birth.
   c. occurs when foreign substances stimulate the production of antibodies.
   d. develops as a result of antibodies that are innate to the organism being stimulated to produce WBCs.

2. When there is cellular injury, which of the following WBCs arrive first and begin phagocytosis?
   a. Lymphocytes.
   b. Basophils.
   c. Monocytes.
   d. Neutrophils.

3. Interleukins

    a. stimulate B lymphocyte activity.

    b. interfere with multiplication of stem cells.

    c. stimulate growth and differentiation of lymphoid cells into lymphocytes.

    d. interfere with the ability of viruses in infected cells to replicate.

4. The function of colony-stimulating factors (CSF) is to

    a. stimulate growth of blood cells.

    b. suppress T-cell production.

    c. inhibit protein production.

    d. stimulate production of antibodies.

5. Natural killer cells act by

    a. releasing powerful chemicals that kill infectious microorganisms.

    b. binding to antigens and damaging their cell membrane.

    c. injecting fluid into the antigen cell, causing edema and death.

    d. decreasing the activities of the B cells.

6. Which of the following immunoglobulins crosses the placenta to provide maternal acquired antibodies to the infant?

    a. IgG.

    b. IgA.

    c. IgM.

    d. IgE.

7. T lymphocyte growth factor (TGF)

    a. promotes wound healing and bone remodeling.

    b. interferes with the multiplication of stem cells.

    c. stimulates the production of erythrocytes.

    d. interferes with the ability of viruses to replicate.

8. A lack of which of the following decreases the number and function of T cells?

    a. Calcium.

    b. Protein.

    c. Potassium.

    d. Fluid volume.

9. Substances that interact with immune cells to induce the immune response are

    a. antigens.

    b. antibodies.

    c. cytokines.

    d. monocytes.

10. Which of the following depresses immune function and increases the risk of developing an infection?

    a. Heart disease.

    b. Use of beta-adrenergic blockers.

    c. Dehydration.

    d. Stress.

43

Immunizing Agents

FILL IN THE BLANKS

Complete the following sentences.

1. Active immunity develops as a result of exposure to an _____ and results in _____. Active immunity may be _____ or _____.

2. Passive immunity occurs when _____ are formed exogenously and transferred to the host. Passive immunity lasts only _____.

3. Vaccines and toxoids are generally contraindicated in persons with _____, _____, or _____, those _____ or _____, and during _____.

4. Tetanus toxoid should be administered every _____ years in adults.

5. The following vaccines are not routinely administered to Americans unless they are traveling abroad:

   a. _____

   b. _____

   c. _____

6. Before you administer a DTP immunization you should check the person's _____.

7. If your client experiences an allergic reaction from the administration of an immunizing agent, _____ should be administered immediately.

8. Persons receiving a DTP injection may experience _____ and _____ at the injection site. They should be instructed to take _____ for symptomatic relief.

9. _____ (_____) is a rare reaction to oral poliovirus vaccine.

10. Urticaria, fever, arthralgia, and enlarged lymph nodes are symptoms of _____, which can occur _____ or _____ after an injection.

EXERCISE ON IMMUNIZATION

Administration of Immunizations

Specify how each immunization is administered.

1. _____ Measles vaccine.

2. _____ Hepatitis B vaccine.

3. _____ Poliovirus vaccine.

4. _____ Tetanus toxoid.

5. _____ Meningitis vaccine.

Schedule for Immunization of Infants and Children

Place an × in the table to identify the appropriate timing(s) for immunizations, based upon recommendations from the Advisory Committee on Immunization Practices (ACIP), the American Academy of Pediatrics (AAP), and the American Academy of Family Physicians (AAFP).

	Birth	1 mo	2 mo	4 mo	6 mo	10–12 mo	15 mo	18 mo	4–6 yr	11–12 yr	Every 10 yr
Polio (OPV)											
Diphtheria–tetanus–pertussis (DTP)											
Diptheria–tetanus (DT)											
Measles–mumps–rubella (MMR)											
Haemophilus influenza Type B (Hib)											
Hepatitis B 1st dose (HBV)											
Hepatitis B 2nd dose (HBV)											
Hepatitis B 3rd dose (HBV)											
HBV, if not previously immunized											
Varicella zoster (Var) chicken pox											

REVIEW QUESTIONS

1. When administering DTP to an 18-month-old, you should give the parents the following instructions:

   a. "Apply cold compresses to the injection site."

   b. "Do not let A.J. walk on her leg for 2 hours."

   c. "Take A.J. home and give her a warm bath and massage her leg."

   d. "Give Tylenol q4–6h because fever is a common adverse reaction to this medication."

2. Persons who have been immunized can develop serum sickness. The symptoms are

   a. laryngeal edema and urticaria.

   b. severe respiratory distress and tachycardia.

   c. fever, arthralgia, and enlarged lymph nodes.

   d. somnolence, convulsions, and dizziness.

3. Mrs. J. tells you that the last time her child received a DTP immunization he had a fever of 104.5°. Identify your nursing actions.

   a. Withhold the immunization and contact the physician.

   b. Administer diphenhydramine hydrochloride (Benadryl) before administration of DTP.

   c. Administer only a DT immunization.

   d. Administer acetaminophen (Tylenol) with the DTP.

4. Mrs. J.'s child has been bitten by a rabid raccoon. Which of these statements leads you to believe that she understands how the rabies vaccine is to be administered?

   a. "My child will receive five IM doses of this drug: one today, then 3 days, 7 days, 14 days, and 28 days later."

   b. "My child must receive a daily injection for 4 weeks."

   c. "My child will receive an initial injection followed by an oral drug for 2 months."

   d. "My child will receive a SC injection every 4 weeks for four doses, then a booster 6 months after the last dose."

5. MMR (measles, mumps, and rubella) vaccination is contraindicated in

   a. persons with lung disease.

   b. persons who have had chicken pox.

   c. children under the age of five.

   d. persons who are pregnant.

6. Drugs that alter the effects of vaccines include

   a. antacids.

   b. corticosteroids.

   c. thiazide diuretics.

   d. beta-adrenergic blockers.

7. Anaphylaxis resulting from the administration of an immunizing agent can be effectively treated with

   a. promethazine hydrochloride (Phenergan).

   b. diphenhydramine hydrochloride (Benadryl).

   c. epinephrine (Adrenalin).

   d. prednisone (Deltasone).

8. Vaccines provide

   a. active immunity.

   b. passive immunity.

   c. natural immunity.

   d. cell-mediated immunity.

9. Vaccines should not be given to children if they

   a. have a febrile illness.

   b. are diabetic.

   c. have a seizure disorder.

   d. weigh less than 20 lb.

10. Mrs. J. asks you why RhoGAM [Rh_0(D) immune globulin] was ordered. The best response would be

    a. "You are an Rh negative mother. If you deliver an Rh positive baby, this medication will prevent Rh_0(D) sensitization."

    b. "You are an Rh positive mother. If you deliver an Rh negative baby, this medication will prevent Rh_0(D) sensitization."

    c. "Because you are an Rh negative mother, you are predisposed to certain infections. This medication prevents you from developing a varicella infection."

    d. "Rh positive mothers are more susceptible to hemorrhage. This immune serum will prevent you from having excessive blood loss."

CRITICAL THINKING CASE STUDY

S., a 6-month-old infant, has come to the clinic to receive her immunizations. Her mother states that S. had a reaction after her last immunization and that she does not want S. to have any more immunizations.

1. Identify what questions you should ask the mother.

2. Identify the information you should give S.'s mother regarding immunizations.

S.'s mother finally agrees to allow the infant to have the immunization.

3. Identify what assessment should be done before administering the DTP and for what reasons you would withhold an immunization.

S.'s mother calls the office to report that S. has a lump on her leg where she received the immunization.

4. Describe the advice you would give S.'s mother.

44

Immunostimulants

MATCHING EXERCISE

Terms and Concepts

Match the concept with the term for it.

1. _____ A drug that stimulates production of RBCs.

2. _____ Stimulates bone marrow to produce WBCs.

3. _____ Decreased production of neutrophils.

4. _____ Used with persons undergoing bone marrow transplantation.

5. _____ Approved for the treatment of Kaposi's sarcoma.

6. _____ Approved for the treatment of renal cell carcinoma.

7. _____ An immunizing agent against tuberculosis, also used for bladder cancer.

8. _____ Normal white blood count.

9. _____ A mood stabilizing agent that mobilizes neutrophils and is sometimes given to persons with chemotherapy-induced neutropenia.

10. _____ A drug that helps restore immunologic function.

A. 5000–10,000/mm^3.

B. Epoetin alfa (Epogen).

C. 15,000–25,000/mm^3.

D. Filgrastim.

E. Bacillus Calmette–Guérin (BCG).

F. Neutropenia.

G. Interleukin-2 (Aldesleukin).

H. Sargramostim.

I. Interferon alpha-2b.

J. Lithium.

K. Levamisole (Ergamisol).

TRUE OR FALSE

1. _____ Interferons can only be administered by injection.

2. _____ Immunostimulants are used exclusively for persons with cancer.

3. _____ Interferons should not be administered to persons who have hepatitis.

4. _____ Toxicity from the administration of interleukin-2 (Aldesleukin) can result in hard to control seizures.

5. _____ Isolation procedures must be instituted if the neutrophil count drops below 500/mm^3.

CROSSWORD PUZZLE

Across

1. Any previous infections should be resolved before beginning therapy with this drug.

3. This type of drug is given only by injection.

4. Low _____ count places the patient at risk of infection.

6. Interferon alpha-n3 is approved only for treatment of recurring _____.

8. Stimulates granulocyte production.

9. An abnormal decrease in white blood cells.

Down

2. Given after bone marrow transplantation via slow IV.

5. Abbreviation for the immunostimulant that can cause bladder cancer remission.

7. This type of tumor in the breast, lung, or colon does not respond to interferon.

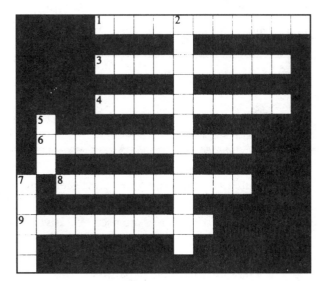

REVIEW QUESTIONS

1. Your client is receiving filgrastim and complains of bone pain. You should

   a. administer a nonsteroidal antiinflammatory drug.

   b. stop the drug immediately.

   c. apply warm compresses to his arms and legs.

   d. assist him with passive range of motion exercises of his extremities.

2. Which of the following drugs, if administered concurrently with aldesleukin, will decrease its effects?

   a. Prednisone.

   b. Propranolol (Inderal).

   c. Ibuprofen (Motrin).

   d. Gentamicin (Garamycin).

3. Which of the following lab studies should be done before initiating immunostimulant drug therapy?

   a. CBC and platelet count.

   b. Creatinine clearance.

   c. Liver function studies.

   d. Electrolytes.

4. The following lab work should be done routinely during immunostimulant therapy:

   a. PT and PTT.

   b. Hematocrit and hemoglobin.

   c. CBC, WBC, and platelet count.

   d. Creatinine clearance.

5. Filgrastim (Neupogen), given to prevent infection in a neutropenic cancer patient, should be initiated

   a. 2 weeks before the initiation of therapy.

   b. within 24 hours after the last dose of a neoplastic agent.

   c. 2 weeks after the initiation of therapy.

   d. throughout the time of the cancer treatment.

6. Interferons help to

   a. normalize white blood counts.

   b. increase hemoglobin levels.

   c. decrease the risk of bleeding.

   d. enhance red blood cell production.

7. Bacillus Calmette–Guérin (BCG), used to treat bladder cancers, is

   a. administered by inhalation.

   b. applied via applicator in gel form.

   c. administered parenterally over 12 hours.

   d. instilled into the bladder.

8. The expected outcome of administering epoetin alfa (Epogen) to a client with chronic renal failure is

   a. decreased bleeding.

   b. increased WBC production.

   c. decreased secretion of renin.

   d. increased RBC production.

9. The administration of sargramostim (Leukine) will

   a. prevent infection.

   b. enhance RBC production.

   c. promote the function of transplanted bone marrow.

   d. prevent rejection of the transplanted bone marrow.

10. A toxic response to aldesleukin can result in

   a. chronically high blood glucose levels.

   b. osteoporosis.

   c. dysrhythmias unresponsive to treatment.

   d. pulmonary fibrosis.

CRITICAL THINKING CASE STUDY

Mr. J., a 36-year-old accountant, is to receive a bone marrow transplant. He will be receiving sargramostim after the procedure to help prevent rejection.

1. Discuss the teaching that you will do with Mr. J. and his wife.

2. Identify the assessments that you will do.

Mr. J. is very nervous after the transplant and asks you when he will know if the graft has been successful and what the possibility of rejection is. (The learner will need additional sources to answer the question below.)

3. Identify how you will respond to Mr. J.'s inquiry.

45

Immunosuppressants

13. _____ Persons receiving methotrexate (Rheuma-trex) should have liver function studies performed monthly.

14. _____ The preferred route for administering cyclosporine (Sandimmune) is parenterally because it is more effective.

15. _____ Symptoms of neurotoxicity produced by cyclosporine include confusion, hallucinations, and seizures.

REVIEW QUESTIONS

1. Mr. P. is receiving methotrexate after a transplant. Methotrexate will also be effective for which one of the following inflammatory disorders that Mr. P. has?
   a. Psoriasis.
   b. Lupus erythematosus.
   c. Acne.
   d. Herpes zoster.

2. Persons receiving azathioprine after a kidney transplant should be observed for
   a. neurotoxicity.
   b. bone marrow depression.
   c. liver toxicity.
   d. renal failure.

3. Your client asks you how corticosteroids work to prevent rejection reactions. The best reply would be
   a. "They decrease formation and function of antibodies and T cells."
   b. "They inhibit the production of neutrophils."
   c. "They reduce the concentration of WBCs."
   d. "They prevent the formation of antigens."

4. A person receiving immunosuppressants should be assessed for graft versus host disease (GVHD). Symptoms include
   a. elevated alkaline phosphatase, transaminase, and bilirubin levels.
   b. a 5–10 point drop in hematocrit and hemoglobin.
   c. peripheral edema and decreased urinary output.
   d. elevated serum potassium, sodium, and calcium levels.

TRUE OR FALSE

1. _____ Rheumatoid arthritis results from an inappropriate activation of the immune response.

2. _____ Acute organ rejection occurs within 2 days following transplantation.

3. _____ Once an individual has had a transplanted organ for a year, he or she will not experience organ rejection.

4. _____ Corticosteroids increase the numbers of circulating basophils, eosinophils, and monocytes.

5. _____ Cytotoxic antimetabolites block cellular reproduction.

6. _____ Methotrexate (Rheumatrex) has been used to treat severe psoriasis.

7. _____ Cyclosporine (Sandimmune) is used to prevent graft versus host disease in transplant recipients.

8. _____ Antithymocyte globulin (ATG) should not be administered to persons who have an allergy to cow serum.

9. _____ Isolation techniques are instituted for transplant recipients whose neutrophil count drops below 1000/mm^3.

10. _____ Immediately following a transplant, the recipient is allowed no visitors to prevent infection.

11. _____ Persons taking immunosuppressants should avoid the use of alcohol and tobacco.

12. _____ Lymphoma may result from immunosuppression.

5. Children receiving corticosteroids to suppress immune reactions need to be told that this can result in

   a. pigmentation changes.

   b. hair loss.

   c. growth retardation.

   d. renal failure.

6. Cushingoid symptoms that can result from long-term administration of corticosteroids include the development of

   a. facial hair.

   b. a buffalo hump.

   c. peripheral edema.

   d. dysrhythmia.

7. Electrolyte deviations associated with long-term administration of corticosteroids for immunosuppression include

   a. hypochloremia.

   b. hypomagnesemia

   c. hypokalemia.

   d. hyponatremia.

8. An adverse effect of immunosuppression is the development of

   a. chronic lung disease.

   b. lupus erythematosus.

   c. ascites.

   d. opportunistic infections.

9. Persons receiving azathioprine (Imuran) should be observed for adverse effects of the drug, including

   a. tachycardia.

   b. peripheral edema.

   c. drop in WBC.

   d. severe diarrhea.

10. K.C. is receiving immunosuppressive agents after a lung transplant. For which one of the following assessments would you contact the physician?

    a. Weight gain of 1½ lb.

    b. Temperature of 37.8°C.

    c. Cough.

    d. Hypoactive bowel sounds.

CRITICAL THINKING CASE STUDY

M.B., a 12-year-old who received a kidney transplant yesterday, is taking cyclosporine (Sandimmune) and prednisone to prevent rejection of the transplanted organ. (The learner may need to use additional sources to answer these questions.)

1. Identify what you will be assessing for and your rationale for each assessment.

2. Describe the adverse effects of these medications.

3. Discuss the teaching that you will do regarding the medications M.B. is taking.

M.B.'s urinary output is minimal and her physician decides to dialyze her. M.B. starts crying, stating, "I've lost my kidney, haven't I?"

4. Describe the best response to M.B.'s statement.

VIII

DRUGS AFFECTING THE RESPIRATORY SYSTEM

46

Physiology of the Respiratory System

MATCHING EXERCISES

Terms and Concepts

Match the concept with the term for it.

1. _____ Hairlike projections that sweep mucus toward the pharynx.

2. _____ The functional units of the lungs.

3. _____ The lining adheres to the surface of the lung.

4. _____ The ability of the lungs to stretch or expand.

5. _____ Regulates the rate and depth of respiration.

6. _____ Stimulates the respiratory center.

7. _____ The normal percentage of oxygen contained in room air.

8. _____ Average tidal volume.

9. _____ Causes bronchodilation.

10. _____ Responsible for carrying O_2.

A. Oxygen level.

B. Carbon dioxide.

C. Visceral pleura.

D. Cilia.

E. Lobules.

F. Medulla oblongata.

G. Pons.

H. 35%.

I. 500 ml.

J. 800 ml.

K. Compliance.

L. Sympathetic nervous system stimulation.

M. 21%.

N. White blood cells.

O. Hemoglobin.

Respiratory System Diagram

Match the letter of the descriptive statement with the corresponding body part in Figure 46-1.

A. Warms and humidifies the air.

B. Where air exchange takes place.

C. Connects the upper and lower respiratory tract.

D. The vocal cords are located here.

E. The walls contain smooth muscle controlled by the autonomic nervous system.

F. This muscle aids in respiration.

G. Mainstem bronchi.

Figure 46-1

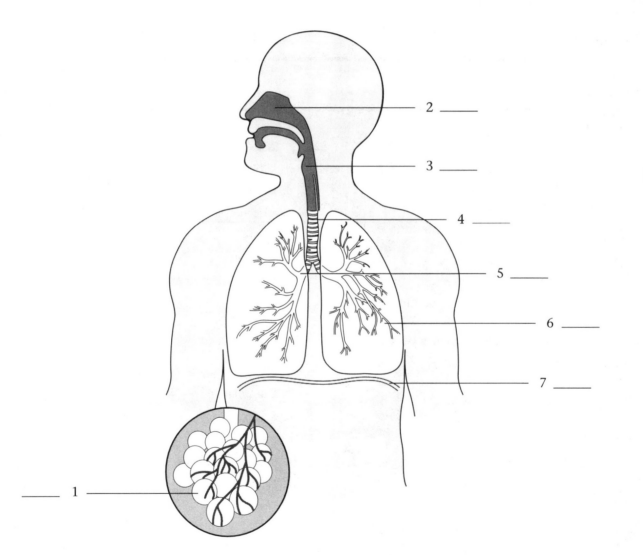

REVIEW QUESTIONS

1. Which of the following causes a decreased respiratory rate?
   a. Fever.
   b. Exercise.
   c. Pain.
   d. Narcotics.

2. Which of the following factors has the most significant impact on diffusion in the lungs?
   a. Lung size.
   b. Pressure differences between gases on each side of the membrane.
   c. Adequate circulation.
   d. The number and depth of respirations per minute.

3. The average number of sighs per hour.
   a. 1–2.
   b. 3–5.
   c. 6–10.
   d. 12–20.

4. The passageway between the upper and lower respiratory tract.
   a. Trachea.
   b. Bronchioles.
   c. Alveoli.
   d. Bronchi.

5. Which is one of the common signs and symptoms of respiratory disorders?
   a. Fever.
   b. Cyanosis.
   c. Hypertension.
   d. Cough.

6. You would document the breathing pattern of a person with a respiratory rate of 30 as
   a. normopnea.
   b. tachypnea.
   c. bradypnea.
   d. apnea.

7. An average tidal volume is
   a. 100 cc.
   b. 250 cc.
   c. 500 cc.
   d. 1000 cc.

8. Which of the following transports O_2 and CO_2?
   a. Hemoglobin.
   b. Albumin.
   c. Leukocytes.
   d. Lymphocytes.

9. Which of the following is responsible for bronchoconstriction?
   a. Parasympathetic nervous system.
   b. Sympathetic nervous system.
   c. Medulla oblongata.
   d. Cerebrum.

10. Cilia
   a. filter air.
   b. secrete mucus.
   c. mobilize mucus.
   d. humidify incoming air.

47

Bronchodilating and Antiasthmatic Drugs

MATCHING EXERCISE

Match the drugs with their effects.

1. _____ Bronchodilators that also have a mild diuretic effect.
2. _____ Reduce intracellular GMP, a bronchoconstricting substance.
3. _____ Reduce inflammation and mucus secretion.
4. _____ Stimulate receptors in bronchial smooth muscle to produce bronchodilation.

A. Adrenergics.

B. Xanthines.

C. Anticholinergics.

D. Corticosteroids.

FILL IN THE BLANKS

Complete the following sentences.

1. Bronchoconstriction may be precipitated by
   a. _____
   b. _____
   c. _____
   d. _____
   e. _____
   f. _____
   g. _____

   h. _____
   i. _____

2. Epinephrine (_____) is administered for an _____. The therapeutic effects will be seen in _____.

3. Albuterol (_____) can be administered _____ or by _____.

4. Ipratropium bromide (_____) improves pulmonary function within _____ minutes. The common adverse effects seen with this drug are _____, _____, _____, _____, _____, and _____.

5. Beclomethasone (_____) (_____) and triamcinolone (_____) are corticosteroids and are administered by _____.

6. Cromolyn (_____) is effective in preventing _____ and _____.

7. Early signs of hypoxia include _____, _____, _____, _____, and _____.

8. Clients with COPD should drink _____ ml/day to _____. They should also avoid excessive caffeine because this may increase _____ and _____.

9. If you are administering two inhalers, a bronchodilator and a corticosteroid, the one you should give first is the _____.

10. After inhalation of a corticosteroid, the client should rinse his or her mouth. This will help prevent a _____.

TRUE OR FALSE

1. _____ Children require a lower dose of theophylline.

2. _____ Cigarette smokers require a higher dose of theophylline than nonsmokers.

3. _____ The physician needs to know the body weight of the client before the correct dosage of theophylline can be determined.

4. _____ Theophylline can cause bradycardia.

5. _____ If an individual has heart failure, a higher dose of theophylline may be required.

REVIEW QUESTIONS

1. Your client may need to have his dosage of theophylline decreased if he
   a. uses insulin.
   b. takes cimetidine (Tagamet).
   c. exercises strenuously.
   d. drinks large amounts of caffeine.

2. You know that your teaching has been successful if your client, who is using beclomethasone (Vanceril), states
   a. "I will limit my intake of caffeine."
   b. "I may gain weight as a result of taking this medication."
   c. "Nausea and vomiting are common adverse effects of this medication, so I will always take it with meals."
   d. "I will rinse my mouth after each use of my inhaler."

3. Which of the following statements by your client leads you to believe that she has understood the teaching you have done regarding cromolyn (Intal)?
   a. "If my weight increases I will need to increase the amount of medication I am taking."
   b. "I can expect to have severe coughing after taking this medication."
   c. "I will need to use a nasal decongestant along with this medication."
   d. "If I do not obtain a therapeutic response from the drug in a month my physician will discontinue it."

4. An expected outcome after the administration of bronchodilators is all of the following *except*
   a. decreased dyspnea.
   b. decreased respiratory rate.
   c. decreased anxiety.
   d. decreased secretions.

5. You should instruct a person started on an ipratropium bromide (Atrovent) inhaler about the common adverse effects of this medication, which include
   a. throat irritation.
   b. bradycardia.
   c. insomnia and anorexia.
   d. headache and gastrointestinal upset.

6. The physician orders ipratropium bromide (Atrovent), albuterol (Proventil), and beclomethasone (Vanceril) inhalers for Mr. P. t.i.d. You should
   a. Question the order; three inhalers should not be given at one time.
   b. Administer the bronchodilators first at 5-minute intervals followed by the steroid 5 minutes later.
   c. Administer each inhaler at 1-hour intervals.
   d. Administer each inhaler at 30-minute intervals.

7. Mrs. P. has a theophylline level drawn and it is 30 µg/ml. You know that this level is
   a. just below a therapeutic level.
   b. a therapeutic level.
   c. slightly above a therapeutic level.
   d. a toxic level.

8. Mr. H. was admitted to your unit 6 months ago weighing 148 lb. His medications at the time of the admission were Theo-Dur 300 mg t.i.d., digoxin 0.125 mg q.d., and furosemide (Lasix) 20 mg b.i.d. You weigh Mr. H. and discover that over the course of the past 6 months, he has lost 30 lb. What will you do next?
   a. Continue to administer the medications as ordered.
   b. Question the Theo-Dur dose as being too high.
   c. Question the Theo-Dur dose as being too low.
   d. Administer the Theo-Dur every other day.

9. A drug that decreases the effectiveness of bronchodilators.
   a. Phenelzine (Nardil).
   b. Erythromycin (E-Mycin).
   c. Propranolol (Inderal).
   d. Cimetidine (Tagamet).

10. When administering intravenous theophylline ethylenediamine (Aminophylline) to Mrs. G., the nurse should observe her closely for

    a. dysrhythmias.

    b. hypertension.

    c. apnea.

    d. depression.

CRITICAL THINKING CASE STUDY

Jenny, a 12-year-old female, is admitted to the emergency room with an acute asthma attack. She has a 9-year history of asthma and is allergic to animal dander and grasses. She is not aware of any exposure that could have precipitated her attack, but the attack did occur during basketball practice. Jenny states that she had also been "fighting off a cold" for a week. Jenny takes albuterol (Proventil) and ipratropium bromide (Atrovent). The physician starts Jenny on an aminophylline drip and orders methylprednisolone (Solu-Medrol) IV push.

1. Identify what questions you would ask Jenny to elicit more assessment information.

2. Identify why the medications were ordered.

Jenny complains of palpitations.

3. Identify what you will say to Jenny and what nursing actions you will take.

Jenny complains of epigastric pain and her physician starts her on cimetidine (Tagamet).

4. Identify your nursing actions.

48

Antihistamines

A. Promethazine hydrochloride (Phenergan).

B. Methdilazine (Tacaryl).

C. Dimenhydrinate (Dramamine).

D. Drowsiness.

E. Diphenhydramine hydrochloride (Benadryl).

F. Cyproheptadine (Periactin).

G. Chlorpheniramine maleate (Chlor-Trimeton).

H. Azatadine maleate (Optimine).

I. Dimetapp.

J. Hydroxyzine (Vistaril).

K. Headache.

L. Loratidine (Claritin).

M. Dizziness.

N. Nausea and vomiting.

MATCHING EXERCISE

Terms and Concepts

Match the concept with the term for it.

1. _____ Used as an antipruritic in allergic and nonallergic pruritus.

2. _____ Used to prevent motion sickness.

3. _____ May affect blood pressure when given parenterally.

4. _____ Given parenterally for treatment of allergic reactions to blood.

5. _____ A very potent antihistamine that produces significant sedation.

6. _____ Weight gain has been reported in persons taking this drug.

7. _____ Should not be used in persons with asthma.

8. _____ Has antihistamine, antiemetic, antianxiety, and sedative effects.

9. _____ A combination product containing an antihistamine, an adrenergic agent, and other ingredients.

10. _____ An adverse effect of the administration of some antihistamines.

11. _____ A newer antihistamine that does not produce drowsiness.

12. _____ When antihistamines are administered for their antiemetic effect, you should see a decrease in this symptom.

REVIEW QUESTIONS

1. Which of the following statements by Mrs. H. indicates successful teaching concerning promethazine hydrochloride (Phenergan)?

   a. "I can still have my after dinner drink."

   b. "I will eat a diet high in roughage while I am taking this medication."

   c. "I will be careful when driving; this medication could make me drowsy."

   d. "I can take this medication as frequently as I need it."

2. Phenothiazines should be used with caution in individuals who have

   a. seizure disorders.

   b. hypertension.

   c. diabetes mellitus.

   d. prostatic hypertrophy.

3. Which of the following conditions could contraindicate the further use of promethazine hydrochloride (Phenergan)?

   a. Anorexia.

   b. Vomiting.

   c. Nausea.

   d. Photosensitivity.

4. Antihistamines should be used with caution in persons with a history of

   a. hypertension.

   b. thyroid dysfunction.

   c. prostatic hypertrophy.

   d. diabetes mellitus.

5. An expected outcome after the administration of antihistamines for Parkinson's disease.

   a. Increased muscle strength.

   b. Decreased rigidity.

   c. Decreased deep tendon reflexes.

   d. Increased coordination.

6. Which of the following antihistamines is effective in treating pruritus?

   a. Astemizole (Hismanal).

   b. Clemastine fumarate (Tavist).

   c. Hydroxyzine hydrochloride (Atarax).

   d. Cyproheptadine (Periactin).

7. Antihistamines are effective in treating the following allergic reactions:

   a. Pruritus.

   b. Bronchoconstriction.

   c. Tachycardia.

   d. Hypotension.

8. Which of the following antihistamines is effective in treating vertigo?

   a. Trimeprazine tartrate (Temaril).

   b. Methdilazine (Tacaryl).

   c. Cyclizine hydrochloride (Marezine hydrochloride).

   d. Meclizine hydrochloride (Antivert).

9. A newer antihistamine that does not cause drowsiness.

   a. Astemizole (Hismanal).

   b. Diphenylpyraline hydrochloride (Hispril).

   c. Azatadine maleate (Optimine).

   d. Loratidine (Claritin).

10. What instructions should you give Mr. C., age 79, who is starting diphenhydramine hydrochloride (Benadryl)?

    a. "If your nose begins to run, use a nasal spray."

    b. "Constipation is common. Increase the roughage in your diet."

    c. "Decrease your sodium intake while you are using this medication."

    d. "Incontinence is an adverse effect of this medication. Contact your physician if it occurs."

CRITICAL THINKING CASE STUDY

Mrs. J. is a 55-year-old woman recently diagnosed with vertigo. The physician orders meclizine hydrochloride (Antivert). (The learner may need additional sources to answer the questions below.)

1. Discuss with Mrs. J. the reason the medication was ordered and the potential adverse effects.

Mrs. J. is very distressed about her diagnosis and asks you if there are any other medications that will help her.

2. Identify your response.

49

Nasal Decongestants, Antitussives, Mucolytics, and Cold Remedies

FILL IN THE BLANKS

Complete the following sentences.

1. These medications are contraindicated for individuals with narrow-angle glaucoma: _____.

2. Coryza is _____.

3. A prominent symptom of respiratory tract infection is a _____.

4. Nonrespiratory conditions that predispose individuals to secretion retention include _____, _____, and _____.

5. Antitussives are used when a nonproductive cough interferes with _____ and _____.

6. This mucolytic is also used for treatment of acetaminophen overdosage: _____ (_____).

7. Ingredients used in narcotic antitussives include _____, _____, _____, and _____.

8. If nasal decongestants are overused they can cause _____.

9. Nasal decongestants can _____ heart rate and blood pressure.

10. Adverse effects associated with the use of narcotic antitussives include _____, _____, _____, _____, _____, _____, and _____.

11. These medications should not be administered with dextromethorphan: _____.

12. Before instilling nasal decongestants, you should have the patient _____.

13. Nasal decongestants should be administered to infants _____.

14. After administering cough syrups, the patient should avoid eating or drinking for _____.

15. Individuals who require expectorants for congestion should be encouraged to drink _____ daily.

CROSSWORD PUZZLE

Across

1. A nasal decongestant.

5. A nonnarcotic antitussive.

9. Many over the counter decongestants can decrease _____ discharge.

Down

2. A mucolytic.

3. An ingredient found in Dristan.

4. Inflammation of the mucous membrane of the nose.

5. A cold, cough, and allergy remedy.

6. An expectorant.

7. A commonly used medication for colds and cough that contains guaifenesin.

8. Agents that suppress coughing by depressing the respiratory center.

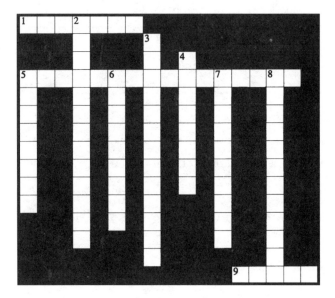

REVIEW QUESTIONS

1. Which statement by your client would lead you to believe that he has understood the instructions you have given him regarding Mucomyst?

   a. "I will blow my nose before instilling the nasal spray."

   b. "I will report any dizziness, drowsiness, or rapid pulse."

   c. "I will drink 2000–3000 ml of fluid daily."

   d. "I will use it only when I am coughing."

2. An adverse reaction commonly experienced by persons using nasal decongestants excessively is

   a. diarrhea and vomiting.

   b. dry mouth.

   c. rash.

   d. rebound nasal congestion.

3. Which of the following statements by your client leads you to believe that he has understood the teaching you have done regarding his expectorant?

   a. "I should increase my intake of fluids."

   b. "It is best to take the medication with meals."

   c. "I should not drive while I am taking this medication."

   d. "I need to lie down for half an hour after I take this medication."

4. Which of the following group of medications, if administered with antitussives, could increase their effects?

   a. Antianxiety agents.

   b. Antihypertensives.

   c. Anticholinergics.

   d. Thiazide diuretics.

5. Which of the following medications would increase the risk of hypertension if administered with nasal decongestants?

   a. Antihistamines.

   b. Thyroid preparations.

   c. Theophylline.

   d. Furosemide (Lasix).

6. Persons taking pseudoephedrine hydrochloride (Sudafed), a nasal decongestant, need to be observed for

   a. respiratory depression.

   b. constipation.

   c. tachycardia.

   d. muscle rigidity.

7. This medication is useful in treating an aceta-minophen overdose.

    a. Acetylcysteine (Mucomyst).

    b. Benzonatate (Tessalon).

    c. Iodinated glycerol (Organidin).

    d. Hydromorphone hydrochloride (Dilaudid).

8. An adverse effect of antitussives is excessive suppression of the cough reflex, which can cause

    a. apnea.

    b. tachypnea.

    c. retained secretions.

    d. increased pH of arterial blood.

9. An expected outcome of the administration of acetylcysteine (Mucomyst) should be

    a. suppression of cough.

    b. decreased nasal discharge.

    c. a productive cough.

    d. decreased respiratory rate.

10. Dr. J. orders 15 drops of 5% organidin solution. How many milliliters will you administer?

    a. 1 ml.

    b. 3 ml.

    c. 5 ml.

    d. 10 ml.

CRITICAL THINKING CASE STUDY

Mr. Z., who has a 10-year history of COPD, has a temperature of 103°. Congestion is audible upon auscultation, and his lung sounds are diminished in the bases bilaterally. The physician orders IV antibiotics, prednisone, saturated solution of potassium iodide (SSKI), and acetylcysteine (Mucomyst). (The learner may need to use additional sources to answer these questions.)

1. Identify the instructions that you will give Mr. Z. before administering the medications.

2. Describe what you will be assessing for.

Mr. Z. has begun coughing up small amounts of tenacious sputum.

3. Identify your nursing actions.

Mr. Z. complains of being nauseated.

4. Identify your nursing actions.

5. Identify the instructions you will give Mr. Z. that may help prevent a recurrence of pneumonia.

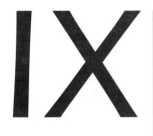

IX

DRUGS AFFECTING THE CARDIOVASCULAR SYSTEM

50

Physiology of the Cardiovascular System

Terms and Concepts

Match the concept with the term for it.

1. _____ Membrane lining the heart chambers.

2. _____ The pacemaker of the heart.

3. _____ Responsible for increasing the heart rate.

4. _____ The smooth inner lining of an artery.

5. _____ Where the exchange of gases, nutrients, and waste products takes place.

6. _____ Helps maintain colloid osmotic pressure.

7. _____ Transports oxygen.

8. _____ Essential to blood coagulation.

9. _____ Functions as a defense mechanism against microorganisms.

10. _____ The resting or filling phase of the cardiac cycle.

A. SA node.

B. Myocardium.

C. Endocardium.

D. Parasympathetic nerves.

E. AV node.

F. Sympathetic nerves.

G. Intima.

H. Leukocytes.

I. Veins.

J. Capillaries.

K. Albumin.

L. Hemoglobin.

M. Diastole.

N. Platelets.

O. Systole.

FILL IN THE BLANKS

Fill in the blanks in Figure 50-1 with the terms below.

Aorta	Pulmonary artery	Left atrium	Left ventricle
Right atrium	Right ventricle	Superior vena cava	Inferior vena cava
Mitral valve	Tricuspid valve	Septum	Chordae tendon
Coronary arteries	Papillary muscle		

Figure 50-1

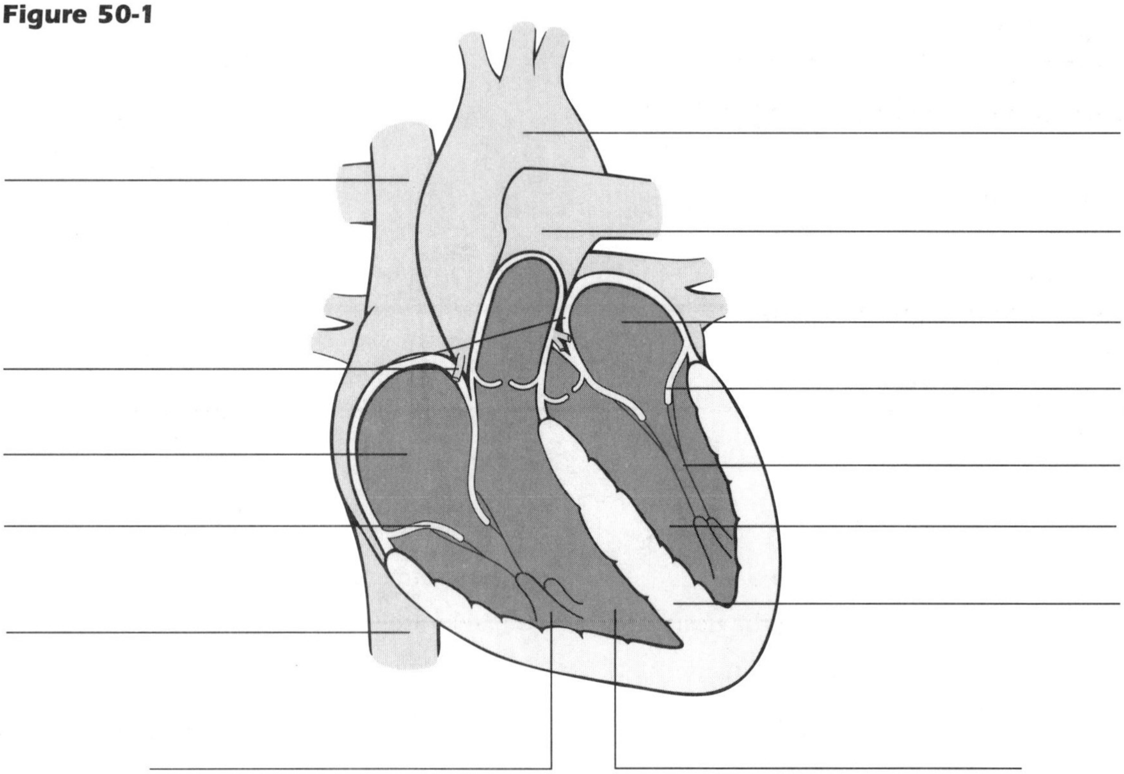

REVIEW QUESTIONS

1. The portion of the heart that receives unoxygenated blood from the vena cava.

   a. Right atrium.

   b. Right ventricle.

   c. Left atrium.

   d. Left ventricle.

2. The valve that separates the right atrium and right ventricle.

   a. Mitral valve.

   b. Tricuspid valve.

   c. Pulmonic valve.

   d. Aortic valve.

3. The ventricles can beat independently at a rate of

   a. 10–20 beats per minute.

   b. 30–40 beats per minute.

   c. 50–60 beats per minute.

   d. 70–80 beats per minute.

4. These vessels carry lymphocytes and large molecules of protein and fat.

   a. Capillaries.

   b. Lymphatic vessels.

   c. Collateral circulation.

   d. Arterioles.

5. This plasma protein helps maintain colloid osmotic pressure.

    a. Fibrinogen.

    b. Gamma globulin.

    c. Leukocyte.

    d. Albumin.

6. This blood component is responsible for transporting oxygen.

    a. Reticulocytes.

    b. Platelets.

    c. Hemoglobin.

    d. Leukocytes.

7. Platelets are produced in the

    a. pancreas.

    b. adrenal glands.

    c. bone marrow.

    d. liver.

8. What percentage of plasma is water?

    a. 25%.

    b. 50%.

    c. 70%.

    d. 90%.

9. An increase in peripheral vascular resistance will

    a. increase blood pressure.

    b. decrease blood pressure.

    c. have no impact on blood pressure.

    d. make blood pressure harder to measure accurately.

10. Blood functions in all of the following ways *except*

    a. transporting oxygen to the cells and carbon dioxide from cells.

    b. carrying leukocytes and antibodies to sites of injury.

    c. producing components necessary for blood coagulation.

    d. regulating body temperature by transferring heat produced by cell metabolism to the skin.

51

Cardiotonic–Inotropic Agents Used in Congestive Heart Failure

FILL IN THE BLANKS

Complete the following sentences.

1. When cardiac output falls, the body attempts to compensate by increasing sympathetic activity, which _____ the force of the contraction, _____ the heart rate, and causes _____. Aldosterone is released and causes increased reabsorption of sodium and water, which _____ blood volume and _____ blood pressure, resulting in _____.

2. As a result of these compensatory mechanisms, there is increased _____ and increased afterload.

3. Digitalis glycosides _____ myocardial contractility and _____ the rate of ventricular contraction.

4. Digitalis is used to treat atrial tachyarrhythmias such as atrial _____, atrial _____, and paroxysmal atrial tachycardia or supraventricular tachycardia.

5. An oral digitalizing dose in an adult is _____ in 24 hours.

6. A child, age 2, weighing 22 lb, requires digitalization. The physician orders 0.04 mg/kg in four equal doses. How much medication will the child receive per dose? _____.

7. Kelly, a newborn who weighs 5 lb and has tetralogy of Fallot, is started on 0.025 mg/kg of digoxin. How much medication will the child receive per day? _____.

8. Amrinone (_____) can be used for _____ management of heart failure not controlled by digitalis and diuretic therapy.

9. When persons are taking digoxin, hypokalemia may precipitate _____.

10. The intravenous dosage of digoxin should be _____ less than the oral dose.

11. Hypomagnesemia (<1.5–2.5 mg/100 ml) leads to _____.

12. Hypercalcemia (>8.5–10 mg/100 ml) enhances _____.

13. Hypokalemia, hypomagnesemia, and hypercalcemia increase the risk of _____.

14. Toxic effects of digitalis include
    a. _____
    b. _____
    c. _____
    d. _____

15. Factors contributing to digoxin toxicity are
    a. _____
    b. _____
    c. _____
    d. _____

MATCHING EXERCISE

Terms and Concepts

Match the concept with the term for it.

1. _____ A heart rate below 60.

2. _____ A complication of acute heart failure characterized by a buildup of secretions in the lungs and respiratory difficulty.

3. _____ The usual daily maintenance dose of digoxin.

4. _____ Administration of relatively large doses of digoxin.

5. _____ A drug used to treat digitalis-induced bradycardia.

6. _____ An electrolyte deviation that can increase the risk of digoxin toxicity.

7. _____ An arrhythmia in which the atrial heart rate is faster than the ventricular rate.

8. _____ An antidote for digitalis toxicity.

9. _____ A K-losing diuretic often used in the treatment of congestive heart failure.

10. _____ The route of digoxin administration used least often because it causes tissue irritation.

11. _____ A therapeutic digoxin level.

A. Digitalization.

B. Oral.

C. Premature ventricular contractions (PVCs).

D. Digoxin immune fab (Digibind).

E. Atropine.

F. Bradycardia.

G. Hypercalcemia.

H. Pulmonary edema.

I. Intramuscular.

J. Furosemide (Lasix).

K. 0.125–0.25 mg.

L. 0.5–2.0 ng/ml.

M. Atrial fibrillation.

N. Tachycardia.

REVIEW QUESTIONS

1. When administering amrinone (Inocor), you should observe for the following adverse effect:

   a. Hyperglycemia.

   b. Thrombocytopenia.

   c. Hypertension.

   d. Convulsions.

2. An expected outcome associated with the administration of digoxin.

   a. Increased heart size.

   b. Increased heart rate.

   c. Decreased edema.

   d. Decreased blood pressure.

3. Persons taking digoxin and verapamil (Calan) concurrently may experience

   a. hyperglycemia.

   b. bradycardia.

   c. hypertension.

   d. convulsions.

4. A drug used for treatment of digoxin toxicity.

   a. Potassium chloride.

   b. Propranolol (Inderal).

   c. Regitine (Phentolamine).

   d. Digoxin immune fab (Digibind).

5. When given with digoxin, which of the following medications will decrease the effect of digoxin?

   a. Isoproterenol (Isuprel).

   b. An antacid.

   c. Furosemide (Lasix).

   d. Epinephrine (Adrenalin).

6. Your client is admitted with acute heart failure and is to be started on digoxin. Which of the following conditions would necessitate an alteration in the drug dose?

   a. Parkinson's disease.

   b. Liver disease.

   c. Impaired renal function.

   d. Diabetes mellitus.

7. Factors that predispose persons to digitalis toxici-

ty include

   a. hyperthyroidism.

   b. hypernatremia, hypermagnesemia, and hypocalcemia.

   c. hypokalemia, hypomagnesemia, and hypercalcemia.

   d. concurrent use of phenytoin (Dilantin).

8. Mr. J. has a serum digoxin level drawn and it comes back 0.4 ng/ml. You know that this is

   a. below the therapeutic level.

   b. a therapeutic level.

   c. above the therapeutic level.

   d. a toxic level.

9. Mrs. P,. who is taking digoxin (Lanoxin) 0.25 mg qd, furosemide (Lasix) 40 mg b.i.d., and potassium 20 mEq b.i.d., states, "What a lovely yellow blouse you are wearing this morning." Your blouse is white. What do you do?

   a. Evaluate Mrs. P. for other symptoms of digoxin toxicity.

   b. Withhold her furosemide (Lasix).

   c. Administer the medication as ordered. Mrs. P. is joking.

   d. Call her physician and ask for additional potassium supplement.

10. S.J. weighs 44 lb and is to be digitalized. The digitalizing dose is to be 0.03 mg/kg in three divided doses. How much will she receive per dose?

   a. 0.2 mg.

   b. 0.3 mg.

   c. 0.4 mg.

   d. 0.6 mg.

CRITICAL THINKING CASE STUDY

M., a 6-year-old weighing 42 lb, is admitted to your unit for treatment for heart failure. She is to be started on digoxin (Lanoxin), furosemide (Lasix), and potassium. The physician orders daily CBCs, digoxin levels, weights, and q4h vital signs.

1. Describe the digitalizing regimen to M.'s mother and tell her what she can expect.

2. Identify the adverse effects you plan to discuss with M.'s mother and why this information is important for her to know.

3. Describe the potential drug interactions you will discuss with M.'s mother.

M.'s mother asks why so many tests are being performed.

4. Explain the reason for the tests in terms both mother and child can understand.

6. Identify and prioritize three nursing diagnoses for a child with heart failure.

5. Identify ways of assessing compliance.

52

Antiarrhythmic Drugs

MATCHING EXERCISE

Terms and Concepts

Match the concept with the term for it.

1. _____ Irregular heart rate or rhythm.

2. _____ Normal cardiac cycle.

3. _____ Time during the cardiac cycle when the heart is unable to respond to a new stimulus.

4. _____ The normal pacemaker of the heart.

5. _____ An abnormal pacemaker.

6. _____ A life-threatening arrhythmia.

7. _____ May indicate impending heart block or cardiovascular collapse.

8. _____ A sign of increased cardiac output.

9. _____ A prolonged PR interval.

10. _____ Symptoms of induced heart failure.

A. Sinus rhythm.

B. Arrhythmia or dysrhythmia.

C. Fatigue and weight gain.

D. First-degree heart block.

E. Increased urinary output.

F. Refractory period.

G. SA node.

H. AV node.

I. Second-degree heart block.

J. Ectopic focus.

K. Tachycardia.

L. Bradycardia.

M. Ventricular fibrillation.

CROSSWORD PUZZLE

Across

9. Drug used to treat atrial fibrillation.

10. Urinary retention can occur with administration of this drug.

Down

1. This medication should be administered with food to prevent GI upset.

2. Slows the ventricular rate; contraindicated in heart failure.

3. This drug is used to treat PVCs when lidocaine is ineffective.

4. For short-term treatment of ventricular arrhythmias.

5. A drug used for long-term treatment of tachyarrhythmias.

6. Used to treat bradycardia.

7. Rapid-acting drug given intravenously for supraventricular tachycardia.

8. Used to treat supraventricular tachycardia, atrial fibrillation, and atrial flutter.

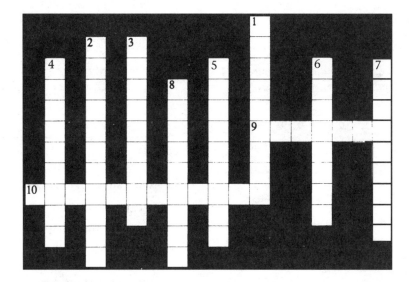

CARDIAC ELECTROPHYSIOLOGY EXERCISE

Part I: Diagram Completion

Fill in the blanks in Figure 52-1 with the terms below to identify the components of the heart's conduction system.

Left ventricle	Left atrium	Right ventricle	Right atrium
Purkinje fibers	Bundle of His	Left bundle branch	Right bundle branch
SA node	AV node		

Figure 52-1

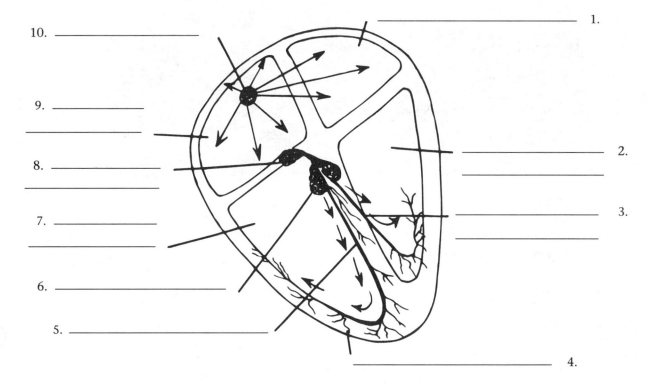

Part II: Drug Effects on Cardiac Physiology

Use the numbers associated with the diagram from Part I of this exercise to complete the following sentences.

1. Pronestyl is used for treating serious refractory dysrhythmias originating in these heart chambers: _____ and _____.

2. Verapamil, a calcium channel blocker, is used to treat supraventricular tachycardia and atrial fibrillation and flutter because it slows conduction through the _____ and _____.

3. Atropine is the drug of choice for heart block because it improves conduction through the _____, and increases conduction through these parts of the heart:

   _____, _____,

   _____, _____

   and _____.

4. Disopyramide (Norpace), given orally to adults to treat ventricular tachyarrhythmias, works by reducing automaticity in the _____ node, slowing conduction through the _____ node, and prolonging the refractory period.

DYSRHYTHMIA ANALYSIS

Select the appropriate term from the list below to pair each of the dysrhythmias with a drug that might be ordered for its treatment.

Digoxin (Lanoxin) Adenosine (Adenocard) Atropine
Lidocaine (Xylocaine) Atrial fibrillation Premature ventricular contractions
Supraventricular tachycardia Sinus bradycardia

1. Dysrhythmia _____ Treatment _____.

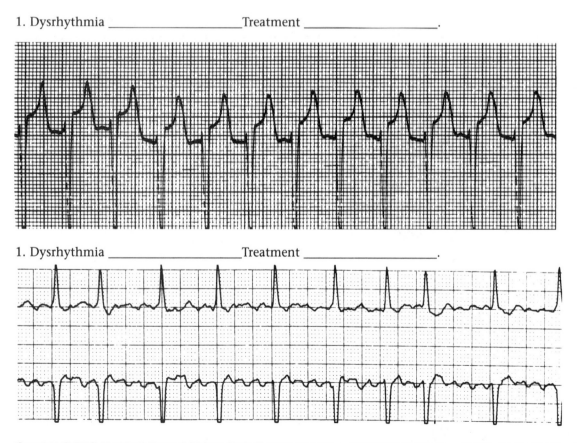

1. Dysrhythmia _____ Treatment _____.

1. Dysrhythmia _____ Treatment _____.

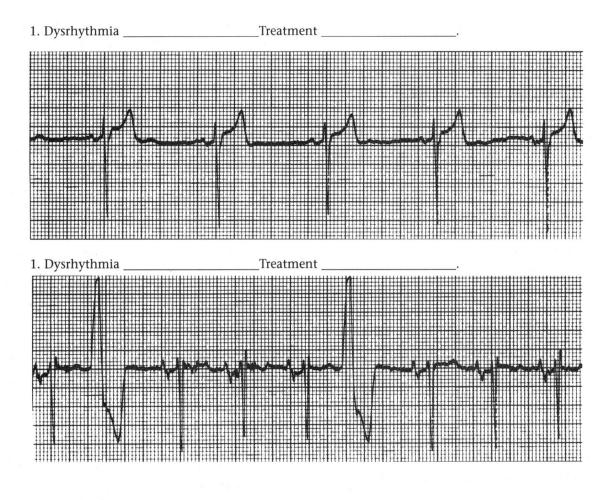

1. Dysrhythmia _____ Treatment _____.

REVIEW QUESTIONS

1. Which of the following conditions would require that the dosage of disopyramide (Norpace) be reduced?

   a. Seizure disorder.

   b. Renal insufficiency.

   c. Hepatotoxicity.

   d. Diabetes mellitus.

2. Side effects of amiodarone (Cordarone) therapy that the nurse should be observing for include

   a. hypotension.

   b. hallucinations.

   c. excessive bruising.

   d. cyanosis.

3. You find your client's IV drip of lidocaine running at 5 mg/minute. You know that this is

   a. below the therapeutic range.

   b. within the therapeutic range.

   c. above the therapeutic range.

   d. a highly toxic range.

4. The following medication may be effective in treating PVCs that are refractory to lidocaine:

   a. Esmolol (Brevibloc).

   b. Bretylium (Bretylol).

   c. Verapamil (Calan).

   d. Adenosine (Adenocard).

5. Persons taking disopyramide (Norpace) should be observed for

   a. paralytic ileus.

   b. urinary retention.

   c. asthma.

   d. diarrhea.

6. The antidysrhythmic agent that is contraindicated for persons with severe uncompensated heart failure is

   a. phenytoin (Dilantin).

   b. quinidine.

   c. lidocaine (Xylocaine).

   d. digoxin (Lanoxin).

7. Your client asks you why he must take quinidine once he gets home. Your best response would be

   a. "Ventricular dysrhythmias can lead to the formation of thrombi on the atria."

   b. "Ventricular dysrhythmias will result in the ventricles beating independently."

   c. "Ventricular dysrhythmias may result in death."

   d. "Ventricular dysrhythmias can cause edema in your extremities."

8. An expected outcome after the administration of antidysrhythmia drugs is increased cardiac output, signs of which include

   a. no complaints of lethargy.

   b. adequate urinary output.

   c. a pulse rate above 80.

   d. no dyspnea.

9. Which of the following drugs, if administered with propranolol (Inderal), will decrease its effects?

   a. Atropine sulfate.

   b. Furosemide (Lasix).

   c. Chloramphenicol (Chloromycetin).

   d. Digoxin (Lanoxin).

10. The physician has ordered 1 gram of lidocaine (Xylocaine) in 500 cc D5W to run at 1 mg/minute. Using micro drip tubing, 1 cc = 60 gtt. How fast will you run the IV to deliver the correct amount of medication?

    a. 15 gtt/minute.

    b. 30 gtt/minute.

    c. 45 gtt/minute.

    d. 60 gtt/minute.

CRITICAL THINKING CASE STUDY

Mr. J., a 56-year-old male weighing 195 lb, is admitted to your unit with a diagnosis of myocardial infarction. You have standing orders in ICU that permit the use of lidocaine (Xylocaine) for treatment of six or more PVCs per minute.

1. Identify how much lidocaine you will administer as a bolus and how much you will use as a maintenance infusion.

Mr. J. continues to have multifocal PVCs that are uncontrolled by lidocaine.

2. Discuss alternatives to the present treatment and your nursing responsibilities.

Mr. J.'s PVCs have resolved, and you are preparing to send him to the cardiac catheterization lab. His EKG shows a PR interval of 0.24 seconds. His heart rate is 60 and BP 106/68.

3. It is time for Mr. J.'s propranolol (Inderal). In light of your observations, discuss what your actions will be.

Mr. J. is preparing for discharge and expresses concerns about resuming an active sex life and asks if the Inderal will affect it. (The student may need to use additional sources to answer this question).

4. Discuss your response to Mr. J.

53

Antianginal Drugs

FILL IN THE BLANKS

Complete the following sentences.

1. Nitrates work by reducing _____ and _____ and decreasing _____ and _____, which decreases _____ and _____. Nitrates increase blood _____ and lower _____.

2. Beta blockers reduce _____ and _____, _____, _____, and _____.

3. Calcium channel blockers dilate _____ and _____, decrease _____, and the conduction system is depressed.

4. Persons who have angina should avoid _____, _____, and _____.

5. Lifestyle changes that will help angina include _____, _____, and exercise.

6. Persons experiencing angina may take nitroglycerin, one every _____ minutes for a maximum of _____ doses. If the pain is unrelieved they should _____.

7. Adverse effects from nitroglycerin include _____, _____, and _____.

8. A person receiving beta-blockers should be observed for _____, _____, _____, and _____.

9. Indicate adverse effects from administration of calcium channel blockers by placing an × next to the appropriate terms:

   a. ____ Heart failure.
   b. ____ Headache.
   c. ____ Diarrhea.
   d. ____ Weakness.
   e. ____ Anorexia.
   f. ____ Confusion.
   g. ____ Nausea.
   h. ____ Bradycardia.

10. If dizziness occurs after administration of antianginal drugs, the client should _____ and _____.

MATCHING EXERCISE

Terms and Concepts

Match the concept with the term for it.

1. _____ A drug used for the long-term treatment of chronic stable angina.

2. _____ A calcium channel blocker used for angina and hypertension.

3. _____ A drug used for the treatment of supraventricular tachycardias.

4. _____ Onset of action of this drug is 1–3 minutes.

5. _____ A common adverse effect of antianginal drugs.

6. _____ This group of drugs is contraindicated in persons with congestive heart failure.

7. _____ A beta-adrenergic blocker given to prevent exercise-induced tachycardia.

8. _____ This group of drugs, when administered with antianginals, will decrease their effects.

9. _____ Tachycardia may occur with administration of this drug.

10. _____ This drug, when given with antianginal drugs, will increase their effects.

A. Nitroglycerin.

B. Nicardipine (Cardene).

C. Anticholinergic drugs.

D. Hypertension.

E. Erythrityl tetranitrate (Cardilate).

F. Nifedipine (Procardia).

G. Verapamil (Calan).

H. Beta-adrenergic blockers.

I. Hypotension.

J. Calcium channel blockers.

K. Propranolol (Inderal).

L. Cimetidine (Tagamet).

FILL IN THE BLANKS

Effects of Nitroglycerin

NITROGLYCERIN

1. Dilation of _____

2. Dilation of _____

3. ↓ _____

4. ↓ _____

5. ↓ _____

↑ Blood supply

6. ↓ _____

7. ↓ _____

8. ↓ _____

REVIEW QUESTIONS

1. The following complaint would indicate that Mr. J. is experiencing an adverse reaction to the nifedipine (Procardia).

   a. "All of my joints ache."

   b. "I have been having severe headaches."

   c. "I have been having trouble breathing."

   d. "My ankles swell a lot, especially at the end of the day."

2. Which of the following instructions should you give your client, who is starting on nitroglycerin?

   a. "Once you get a headache, take no more medication because a therapeutic level has been reached."

   b. "You can take as much nitroglycerin as you need to control the pain."

   c. "If you become dizzy when you take the nitroglycerin, do not take any more."

   d. "You can take up to three tablets at 5-minute intervals. If you do not get relief go directly to the hospital."

3. Which of the following instructions should be included in the discharge teaching for a client discharged with a transdermal nitroglycerin patch?

   a. "Apply the patch to the front of the chest around the heart."

   b. "Apply the patch at the same time each day."

   c. "If you get a headache, apply the patch below your elbows or knees."

   d. "Apply a thin layer of cream to your skin before you apply the patch to avoid irritation."

4. A client, admitted with unstable angina, is started on a nitroglycerin patch and sublingual nitroglycerin. He asks you why both medications were ordered. Your best response would be

   a. "If your physician used only one medication, he would have to use a larger dose which could cause you to have an adverse reaction."

   b. "The patch is for long-term prevention and the sublingual medication is for acute attacks."

   c. "It is very unusual for a physician to order two nitrates. I will speak to your physician."

   d. "If only a patch were used, such large doses would be required that skin irritation may result."

5. Your client has a history of alcohol abuse, hypertension, malnutrition, and asthma. What factors should the nurse take into consideration when a beta-adrenergic blocking agent is ordered for his angina?

   a. A person who ingests alcohol will require larger amounts of a beta-adrenergic blocker.

   b. Low serum albumin levels that result from malnutrition make it necessary to lower the dosage of beta-adrenergic blockers.

   c. Beta-adrenergic blockers are contraindicated for persons with asthma.

   d. Beta-adrenergic blockers may increase blood pressure.

6. Nitrates relieve angina pain by reducing afterload, which is

   a. blood volume within the heart.

   b. pressure within the heart.

   c. peripheral vascular resistance.

   d. oxygen demand of the heart.

7. Beta-adrenergic blocking agents help relieve angina by

   a. reducing oxygen demand of the heart.

   b. increasing the heart rate.

   c. increasing the blood pressure.

   d. reducing circulatory blood volume.

8. Your client is started on intravenous nitroglycerin. You should be observing him for

   a. hypotension.

   b. bronchospasm.

   c. congestive heart failure.

   d. ventricular arrhythmias.

9. Which of the following drugs, if administered with antianginal drugs, will decrease their effects?

   a. Promethazine (Phenergan).

   b. Digoxin (Lanoxin).

   c. Cimetidine (Tagamet).

   d. Isoproterenol (Isuprel).

10. Mrs. A. is taking atenolol (Tenormin) for angina, and you find that her pulse is 54. What should you do?

    a. Tell Mrs. A. to stop taking the medication and reassess her pulse the next day.

    b. Tell Mrs. A. to stop taking the medication and discuss it with her physician at her next appointment.

    c. Contact Mrs. A.'s physician and request that the medication be tapered.

    d. Instruct Mrs. A. to continue to take the medication as ordered.

CRITICAL THINKING CASE STUDY

Mr. D. comes to the emergency room complaining of severe chest pain. Three years ago his physician prescribed nadolol (Corgard) for hypertension, which he stopped taking last year because of sexual dysfunction. The physician starts a nitroglycerin drip.

1. Identify what assessments you will make during the infusion of the nitroglycerin.

Once Mr. D. has stabilized he is started on diltiazem (Cardizem).

2. Explain the rationale for the choice of this drug to treat Mr. D.'s angina.

3. Identify the side effects of the drug that you will discuss with Mr. D.

Mr. D.'s physician also orders a nitroglycerin patch, which is to be put on at 6 A.M. and taken off at 10 P.M.

4. Explain to the client why he is to use the patch in this way and what the potential side effects are.

54

Drugs Used in Hypotension and Shock

TRUE OR FALSE

1. _____ Alkalosis may decrease the effectiveness of dopamine (Intropin).

2. _____ Dobutamine (Dobutrex) will decrease cardiac output.

3. _____ When small doses of dopamine are administered, the client may experience hypotension.

4. _____ Epinephrine (Adrenalin) can produce ventricular arrhythmias and reduce renal blood flow.

5. _____ Isoproterenol (Isuprel) decreases the heart rate and increases diastolic blood pressure.

6. _____ If extravasation of dopamine (Intropin) or levarterenol (Levophed) occurs, severe tissue damage can result.

7. _____ Dopamine (Intropin), dobutamine (Dobutrex), and isoproterenol (Isuprel) can be administered orally or parenterally.

8. _____ Vasopressors can increase oxygen consumption and produce myocardial ischemia.

9. _____ Beta-adrenergic blockers administered concurrently with vasopressors increase effects of the vasopressor agents.

10. _____ Adequate fluid therapy is necessary for dopamine (Intropin) to be effective.

FILL IN THE BLANKS

Complete the following sentences.

1. Common symptoms of shock include _____ urinary output, _____ cardiac output, _____ orientation, seizures, cool extremities, and coma.

2. Drugs with alpha-adrenergic activity increase _____.

3. Drugs with beta-adrenergic activity increase _____ and _____.

4. When you are treating someone for shock, you want to keep their blood pressure above _____, their heart rate below 100, and their urinary output above _____.

5. The drug of choice for treating extravasation is _____ (_____).

REVIEW QUESTIONS

1. Vasopressor drugs can increase oxygen consumption and cause
   a. postural hypotension.
   b. chest pain.
   c. confusion.
   d. abdominal distention.

2. This nursing diagnosis would take priority when caring for a client with anaphylactic shock.
   a. Altered tissue perfusion.
   b. Altered comfort.
   c. Risk for injury.
   d. Altered bowel elimination.

3. The doctor has ordered dopamine (Intropin) to treat your client's hypovolemic shock due to severe blood loss. For the medication to be effective, the physician must also order
   a. fluid replacement.
   b. beta-stimulating drugs.
   c. antibodies.
   d. fluid restriction.

4. An expected outcome after administration of vasopressor drugs is

   a. respiratory rate of 24.

   b. heart rate of 100.

   c. diastolic blood pressure between 80 and 100 mmHg.

   d. urinary output of 30–50 ml/hour.

5. Mr. J. is started on an IV drip of isoproterenol (Isuprel) for hypotension after open heart surgery. What side effect will you be assessing for?

   a. Hypertension.

   b. Tachycardia.

   c. Dyspnea.

   d. Cyanosis.

6. J. has an IV hanging of 200 mg of dopamine (Intropin) in 250 cc of D5W (800 μg/1 cc). If the physician wants J. to receive 160 μg/minute, how fast will you run the IV (use micro drip tubing, 1 cc = 60 gtt)?

   a. 10 gtt/minute.

   b. 12 gtt/minute.

   c. 15 gtt/minute.

   d. 18 gtt/minute.

7. If you note that dopamine (Intropin) has extravasated, you should

   a. administer a beta-adrenergic blocker.

   b. apply a tourniquet.

   c. apply ice and elevate the extremity.

   d. administer phentolamine (Regitine).

8. Which of the following statements by Mr. P. leads you to believe that he has understood the teaching you have done regarding dopamine (Intropin)?

   a. "They will be adjusting this medication frequently to try and regulate my blood pressure."

   b. "I know that they will be monitoring my pulse frequently because it could drop."

   c. "This drug will increase the force of the contraction of my heart."

   d. "The doctor has ordered this medication to increase my heart rate."

9. Which of the following decreases the effectiveness of dopamine (Intropin)?

   a. Acidosis.

   b. Alkalosis.

   c. Hypokalemia.

   d. Hypocalcemia.

10. Beta-stimulating drugs should be used cautiously following a myocardial infarction because they can

   a. increase the peripheral resistance, causing decreased perfusion to the coronary arteries.

   b. decrease myocardial contractility and impair oxygen exchange.

   c. increase oxygen consumption and thereby extend the area of infarction.

   d. raise the blood pressure and therefore stress the heart.

CRITICAL THINKING CASE STUDY

Mr. B. is admitted to the ICU after an MI. He is presently experiencing cardiogenic shock. The physician orders dopamine 200 mg in 250 ml of D5W (Mr. B. weighs 220 lb).

1. Calculate the appropriate number of micrograms Mr. B. should be receiving per minute and identify the assessments that you will perform.

You have been unable to keep Mr. B.'s BP above 80/40, and his urinary output has dropped to 20 cc/hour. The physician decides to add dobutamine (Dobutrex).

2. Identify why Mr. B.'s physician is adding dobutamine (Dobutrex).

Mr. B. begins to experience chest pain. Nitroglycerin is added to his medication regime. Mr. B. has standing orders for O$_2$ and morphine 2 mg. (The student may want to use additional sources to answer this question.)

3. Identify why Mr. B. is experiencing chest pain, and list your nursing actions in order of priority.

55

Antihypertensive Drugs

Terms and Concepts

Match the drug group with its effect.

1. _____ Alpha$_1$ receptor blocking agents.

2. _____ Alpha$_2$ receptor agonist.

3. _____ Beta-adrenergic blocking agents.

4. _____ Calcium channel blocking agents.

5. _____ Diuretics.

6. _____ Vasodilator.

7. _____ ACE inhibitors.

A. Block SNS impulses in the brain.

B. Decrease cardiac output and peripheral resistance.

C. Cause loss of sodium and water.

D. Cause dilation of blood vessels and decreases peripheral resistance; requires concomitant use of a diuretic.

E. Dilate blood vessels and decreases peripheral resistance.

F. Decrease heart rate, force of the contraction, cardiac output, and renin release.

G. Block the enzyme that converts angiotensin I to angiotensin II.

FILL IN THE BLANKS

Cardiovascular Indications for Use

Place an × in the table to identify the appropriate indication(s) for each drug.

	Angina pectoris	Hypertension	Arrhythmias	Heart failure	MI
Amlodipine (Norvasc)					
Enalapril (Vasotec)					
Diltiazem (Cardizem)					
Felodipine (Plendil)					
Nifedipine (Adalat, Procardia)					
Verapamil (Calan, Isoptin)					
Captopril (Capoten)					
Propranolol (Inderal)					
Metoprolol (Lopressor)					
Esmolol (Brevibloc)					

Name That Drug

1. _____ Used to treat neonatal hypertension.

2. _____ A beta blocker that may be used for hypertensive crisis.

3. _____ Commonly used as an IV drip after open heart surgery to maintain the blood pressure within normal limits.

4. _____ A drug used for the treatment of mild hypertension that can cause potassium loss.

5. _____ These are the drugs of choice for persons over 50 with high renin levels.

6. _____ These drugs may be useful for persons who have angina and hypertension.

7. _____ This group of drugs stimulates the sympathetic nervous system, causing fluid retention.

8. _____ Available in a skin patch that can be applied once a week.

9. _____ A nonpharmacologic way of controlling blood pressure.

10. _____ These drugs are effective in treating hypertension for persons with renal disease.

11. _____ These antihypertensive medications produce hyperglycemia, hyperuricemia, and hypercalcemia in adults.

12. _____ Depression is an adverse effect of this medication.

13. _____ Abrupt withdrawal of this drug can cause a hypertensive crisis.

14. _____ ACE inhibitor used once daily for treatment of hypertension.

15. _____ Antihypertensive medications that are only used as step II or higher drugs.

16. _____ Insulin-dependent diabetics may have difficulty controlling their blood sugar if they are placed on this drug to control their blood pressure.

REVIEW QUESTIONS

1. The physician prescribes captopril (Capoten) for Mr. B. You know that Mr. B. needs additional instruction regarding orthostatic hypotension if he says
   a. "If I become dizzy, I will eat something high in sodium."
   b. "I will make sure to rise slowly from a supine position."
   c. "I will not take hot baths and showers."
   d. "I will sleep with the head of my bed elevated."

2. Mrs. H., who is being treated for hypertension, should be instructed to avoid foods high in
   a. vitamin C.
   b. calcium.
   c. potassium.
   d. sodium.

3. Mrs. G. is admitted to the ICU complaining of chest pain. According to Mrs. G., her usual BP is 150/90. On admission, her BP was 170/100. Based on the latest readings, how would you classify Mrs. G.'s blood pressure?
   a. Mild hypertension.
   b. Moderate hypertension.
   c. Severe hypertension.
   d. Hypertensive crisis.

4. The most effective group of antihypertensive drugs for treating hypertension related to high renin levels is
   a. ACE inhibitors.
   b. beta-adrenergic blockers.
   c. calcium channel blockers.
   d. diuretics.

5. The physician orders nitroprusside (Nipride) 50 mg in 250 cc D5W to infuse at 1 μg/kg/min for Mr. J., who weighs 154 lb. How fast will you run the IV (using micro drip tubing, 1 cc = 60 gtt) to deliver the correct amount of medication?
   a. 21 gtt/minute.
   b. 23 gtt/minute.
   c. 25 gtt/minute.
   d. 27 gtt/minute.

6. The following lab value deviation is associated with the use of thiazide diuretics.
   a. Hypoglycemia.
   b. Hypernatremia.
   c. Hypocalcemia.
   d. Hyperuricemia.

7. The following instruction should be given to a client who is started on clonidine (Catapres):
   a. "Take the medication on an empty stomach."
   b. "Have your blood pressure checked daily."
   c. "Do not abruptly stop the medication."
   d. "Check your pulse before taking the medication."

8. For a person with a history of COPD who is experiencing hypertension, the selective beta-adrenergic blocker of choice is
   a. propranolol (Inderal).
   b. nadolol (Corgard).
   c. timolol (Blocadren).
   d. atenolol (Tenormin).

9. Which one of the following complaints may be directly related to reserpine (Serpasil)?
   a. Headache.
   b. Chest pain.
   c. Depression.
   d. Nausea.

10. The following medication may contribute to your client's elevated blood pressure:
    a. Tylenol.
    b. Synthroid.
    c. Oral contraceptives.
    d. Vitamin E.

CRITICAL THINKING CASE STUDY

Your client M. is a 35-year-old female race car driver who weighs 200 lb and smokes two packages of cigarettes per day. Her doctor prescribes atenolol (Tenormin) for her essential hypertension.

1. Identify what lifestyle changes would help M. lower her blood pressure.

2. Identify why this medication was chosen for M.

3. Discuss the teaching you will do with M.

4. Identify ways of promoting compliance.

Three years after her initial treatment for hypertension, M. is seen at the physician's office. Her BP is 150/90 and she has symptoms of chronic renal failure. The physician changes her medication to enalapril (Vasotec) and bumetanide (Bumex).

5. Discuss why M.'s physician ordered two medications at this time.

56

Diuretics

FILL IN THE BLANKS

Complete the following sentences.

1. The nephron functions by three processes:
   _____, _____,
   and _____.

2. A minimum daily urine output of
   _____ is required to remove
   _____ of _____.

3. Most reabsorption occurs in the
   _____.

4. _____ promotes reabsorption
   of _____ from the distal
   tubules and collecting ducts.

5. _____, a hormone from the
   adrenal cortex, promotes
   _____ reabsorption and
   _____ loss.

6. In the proximal tubules _____,
   _____, _____,
   and _____ are secreted.

7. In the distal tubules _____,
   _____, and _____
   are secreted.

8. Edema occurs because of
   a. _____
   b. _____
   c. _____

9. Diuretics are often used for persons with edema
   because they mobilize _____ by
   _____.

10. Diuretics are used for persons with hypertension
    because they decrease _____
    and deplete _____, which may
    _____.

11. _____ are the most frequently
    prescribed diuretic agents. The diuretic effect
    occurs within _____ hours.

12. Potassium-sparing diuretics decrease the exchange of _____ for _____. _____ is the major adverse effect.

13. Osmotic agents increase _____ (_____), which causes _____ to be pulled from extravascular sites into the _____. _____ (Osmitrol) has many uses.

14. Before administering diuretics, the following blood values should be assessed because diuretics can alter these values: _____, _____, _____, _____, and _____.

15. Other assessments the nurse should do when a person is receiving a diuretic include measuring _____, _____, and _____ and assessing for _____.

16. When diuretics are given with digoxin, there is an increased risk of _____ related to _____.

17. A normal serum potassium level is _____.

18. If hypokalemia should occur, it can be treated in the following ways:

    a. _____

    b. _____

    c. _____

    d. _____

    e. _____

19. Hypokalemia can produce the following symptoms:

    a. _____

    b. _____

    c. _____

    d. _____

    e. _____

    f. _____

    g. _____

    h. _____

    i. _____

TRUE OR FALSE

1. _____ Hypoglycemia is a common side effect associated with thiazide administration that can be reversed when diuretic therapy is discontinued.

2. _____ Hyperuricemia can cause gout in persons taking thiazide diuretics.

3. _____ Loop diuretics, when administered rapidly, can cause transient hearing loss.

4. _____ When loop diuretics are administered with aminoglycosides, the effects of the diuretic are decreased.

5. _____ Hypernatremia, hypermagnesemia, and hyperchloremia are common with the long-term use of diuretics.

6. _____ Loop diuretics and potassium-sparing diuretics should not be administered concurrently.

7. _____ The maximum daily dose of furosemide (Lasix) is 100 mg.

8. _____ Diuretics should not be administered to clients in renal failure.

9. _____ Nonsteroidal anti-inflammatory drugs can interfere with the effectiveness of diuretics.

10. _____ Diuretics should be started at a low dosage and gradually increased.

FILL IN THE BLANK

The Nephron

Fill in the blanks in Figure 56-1 with the terms below.

Descending limb of loop of Henle   Glomerulus   Ascending limb of loop of Henle

Loop of Henle   Efferent arteriole   Bowman's capsule

Afferent arteriole   Distal tubule   Collecting tubule

Proximal tubule

Figure 56-1

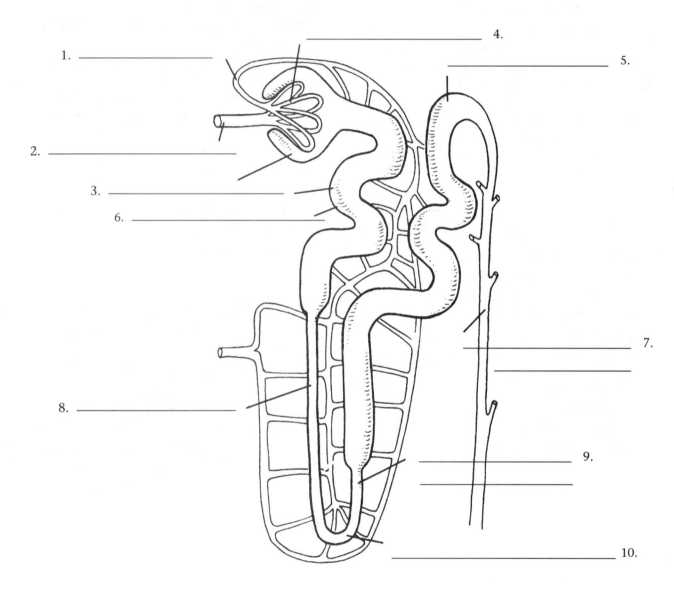

REVIEW QUESTIONS

1. When loop diuretics are administered orally, you can expect to see a response to the medication in
   a. 5 minutes.
   b. 15–20 minutes.
   c. 30–60 minutes.
   d. 2 hours.

2. Miss H. is started on mannitol (Osmitrol) after an automobile accident to decrease her intracranial pressure. This drug works by
   a. promoting retention of sodium and water and excretion of potassium.
   b. blocking the exchange of sodium and potassium at the distal tubules.
   c. raising osmotic pressure, which pulls water from extravascular sites into the bloodstream.
   d. decreasing the reabsorption of chloride, bicarbonate, and sodium at the loop of Henle.

3. Edema is caused by decreased plasma osmotic pressure, which occurs as a result of the loss of
   a. capillary permeability.
   b. sodium.
   c. potassium.
   d. plasma proteins.

4. The following is the most accurate way to assess a person taking diuretics for fluid retention.
   a. Weigh him daily.
   b. Measure his intake and output.
   c. Monitor his vital signs daily.
   d. Assess his electrolytes.

5. The following lab value should be assessed to pick up an adverse response to hydrochlorothiazide (Hydrodiuril).
   a. Sodium levels.
   b. Glucose levels.
   c. Calcium levels.
   d. Chloride levels.

6. Mr. C. has been using a thiazide diuretic for a year, and his serum potassium level is 3.1 mEq/liter. This indicates that
   a. Mr. C. needs a potassium supplement.
   b. the dosage of the diuretic should be decreased.
   c. the dosage of the diuretic should be increased.
   d. the diuretic should be discontinued.

7. Identify why spironolactone (Aldactone) and furosemide (Lasix) are ordered together.
   a. Moderate doses of two different types of diuretics are more effective than a large dose of one type.
   b. This combination promotes diuresis but eliminates hypokalemia.
   c. This combination prevents dehydration and hypovolemia.
   d. Using two drugs increases osmolality of plasma and the glomerular filtration rate.

8. You will check the lab values of your client who has started on furosemide (Lasix) because you know a side effect of this medication is
   a. hyperchloremia.
   b. hypernatremia.
   c. hypokalemia.
   d. hypophosphatemia.

9. The following is a loop diuretic:
   a. Spironolactone (Aldactone).
   b. Bumetanide (Bumex).
   c. Mannitol (Osmitrol).
   d. Hydrochlorothiazide (Hydrodiuril).

10. Your client is admitted to the hospital with pneumonia, and he has a history of chronic renal insufficiency. His physician orders furosemide (Lasix) 40 mg b.i.d. because it
    a. will not cause potassium loss.
    b. is effective in treating persons with pulmonary congestion.
    c. is effective in persons with renal insufficiency.
    d. will increase his pO_2 levels.

CRITICAL THINKING CASE STUDY

Mr. P., a 69-year-old, is admitted with acute heart failure. His physician orders digoxin (Lanoxin) 0.25 mg q.d., furosemide (Lasix) 20 mg b.i.d., and spironolactone (Aldactone) 25 mg b.i.d.

1. Discuss why Mr. P.'s physician ordered these medications.

2. Identify what you should be assessing for (including lab values).

Three days after admission, Mr. P. has lost 10 lb. When you go into his room to do his morning assessment, you find that he is confused.

3. Identify your nursing actions.

57

Anticoagulant, Antiplatelet, and Thrombolytic Agents

Drug Interactions

*Indicate whether the following drugs, when administered concurrently with Coumadin, will **increase** or **decrease** its effects.*

1. _____ Tetracycline.
2. _____ Aspirin.
3. _____ Cholestyramine.
4. _____ Maalox.
5. _____ Cimetidine.
6. _____ Estrogen.
7. _____ Amitriptyline.
8. _____ Synthroid.
9. _____ Lasix.
10. _____ Alcohol.

Drug Indications and Actions

		Heparin	Coumadin	Streptokinase
1.	Indications for use			
2.	Onset			
3.	Duration			
4.	Route			
5.	Blood tests			
6.	Antidote			

REVIEW QUESTIONS

1. The effects of heparin are monitored by this lab test.
   a. CBC.
   b. APTT.
   c. PT.
   d. BUN.

2. Bleeding resulting from the administration of warfarin sodium (Coumadin) should be treated with
   a. Vitamin E.
   b. Vitamin K.
   c. Protamine sulfate.
   d. Calcium gluconate.

3. You know that Mr. J. has understood the teaching regarding anticoagulants if he states
   a. "I can still take over the counter medications if I have a cold."
   b. "I will inform my dentist about my medication before he performs any treatments."
   c. "I will use aspirin for arthritis pain."
   d. "I will continue to play rugby, but I will be careful."

4. Your client's PT is 20 seconds. This is
   a. a lower than therapeutic level.
   b. a higher than therapeutic level.
   c. a therapeutic level.
   d. a dangerously high level.

5. Your client is receiving heparin. After the ABGs are drawn, you should hold his wrist
   a. 1 minute.
   b. 2 minutes.
   c. 4 minutes.
   d. 5 minutes or longer.

6. You know that Mr. C. needs additional teaching about Coumadin if he states
   a. "I will avoid walking barefoot."
   b. "I will not drink alcoholic beverages."
   c. "I will increase the dark green leafy vegetables in my diet."
   d. "I will contact my physician before I take over the counter medications."

7. Which of the following medications, if administered concurrently with warfarin sodium (Coumadin) will increase the risks of bleeding?
   a. Cholestyramine (Questran).
   b. Furosemide (Lasix).
   c. Cimetidine (Tagamet).
   d. Griseofulvin (Fulvicin).

8. You know that your client has a good understanding of why aspirin is being used if he states that aspirin will
   a. inhibit platelet aggregation.
   b. eliminate certain clotting factors.
   c. prevent blood from clotting.
   d. dissolve the clots.

9. You should administer heparin in the
   a. abdomen.
   b. arm.
   c. back.
   d. leg.

10. The physician orders 18,000 U of heparin in 500 cc D5W to be administered over 24 hours. How many units of heparin will the client receive per hour?
    a. 575 units.
    b. 650 units.
    c. 750 units.
    d. 825 units.

CRITICAL THINKING CASE STUDY

M., a 25-year-old female, has been hospitalized with a fractured femur after a motor vehicle accident. M. weighs 200 lb, smokes one package of cigarettes per day, and is taking birth control pills and DiaBeta. M.'s BP is 180/90, pulse 90, and respirations 24 when she is admitted. During the night, she becomes short of breath and complains of chest pain. (Additional sources will be necessary to answer this question.)

1. Identify and prioritize your nursing actions.

The physician diagnoses M. with pulmonary embolism and starts her on a continuous infusion of heparin (1000 units/hour).

2. Discuss why M. was a high risk for developing pulmonary embolism.

M. is started on warfarin (Coumadin) while she is still receiving heparin.

3. Discuss why the two anticoagulants are being given together and identify how the dosage of Coumadin is determined.

58

Antilipemics and Peripheral Vasodilators

Terms and Concepts

Match the drug with its side effects.

1. _____ Cholestyramine (Questran).
2. _____ Gemfibrozil (Lopid).
3. _____ Lovastatin (Mevacor).
4. _____ Nicotinic acid (Niacin).
5. _____ Pentoxifylline (Trental).
6. _____ Isoxsuprine (Vasodilan).

A. Flushing of head and neck.

B. Weakness, muscle cramps, increased angina.

C. Constipation.

D. Headache, skin rash, pruritus.

E. Tachycardia, hypotension, dizziness.

F. Dyspepsia, nausea, vomiting.

FILL IN THE BLANKS

Treatment of Hyperlipidemia

Treatment	Hyperlipidemia					
	I	IIa	IIb	III	IV	V
Cholestyramine (Questran)						
Pravastatin (Pravachol)						
Gemfibrozil (Lopid)						
Nicotinic acid (Niacin)						
Colestipol						
Lovastatin (Mevacor)						
Diet modification						
Exercise						

REVIEW QUESTIONS

1. Your client should be taught to report which of the following adverse effects of pentoxifylline (Trental)?

    a. Blurred vision.

    b. Shortness of breath.

    c. Dizziness and headache.

    d. Diarrhea.

2. Which of the following statements by your client leads you to believe that she understands the teaching you have done regarding cholestyramine (Questran)?

    a. "I will take the medication on an empty stomach."

    b. "I will increase the roughage in my diet."

    c. "I will weigh myself weekly."

    d. "I will have my blood pressure checked weekly."

3. Mrs. J. is started on pentoxifylline (Trental) and complains of nausea. You tell her

    a. "Stop the medication immediately."

    b. "Take the full dose before bedtime."

    c. "Take the medication with meals."

    d. "Continue to take the medication because the nausea will eventually go away."

4. Papaverine (Pavabid) is ordered for your client. An expected outcome is a (an)

    a. decrease in jaundice.

    b. increase in movement of extremities.

    c. decrease in blood pressure.

    d. increase in warmth in her extremities.

5. Hyperlipoproteinemia is caused by this disorder.

    a. Alcoholism.

    b. Diverticulosis.

    c. Hypertension.

    d. Hyperthyroidism.

6. Before Mrs. H. is started on isoxsuprine hydrochloride (Vasodilan), she should be given these instructions.

    a. "You may experience nausea, vomiting, and diarrhea from this medication. It will subside."

    b. "If you experience weakness and severe muscle cramps, don't be alarmed. It is common."

    c. "You will need to increase your intake of yellow vegetables while you are taking this medication."

    d. "You may experience hypotension and dizziness, so move slowly from a sitting position to a standing position."

7. A drug that increases the effects of niacin is

    a. Alcohol.

    b. Insulin.

    c. Prednisone.

    d. Estrogen.

8. Once started on niacin, your client can expect to see a decrease in her cholesterol in

    a. 1 week.

    b. 3–5 weeks.

    c. 2–5 weeks.

    d. 1–3 months.

9. An expected outcome after the administration of pentoxifylline (Trental) is

    a. increased peripheral pulses.

    b. decreased peripheral edema.

    c. increased sensation in all extremities.

    d. decreased leg pain with exercise.

10. Flushing of the face and neck is a common side effect after administration of nicotinic acid (Niacin). The following will decrease the flushing reaction:

    a. Administer niacin with an antacid.

    b. Administer aspirin 30 minutes before nicotinic acid.

    c. Administer diphenhydramine hydrochloride (Benadryl) with the niacin.

    d. Apply cold compresses to the head and neck.

CRITICAL THINKING CASE STUDY

Mr. J., a 55-year-old male, is admitted with leg ulcers and peripheral edema secondary to peripheral vascular disease. He is being evaluated for a bypass graft. His physician orders isoxsuprine hydrochloride (Vasodilan) 20 mg q.i.d. (Students may need to use additional sources to answer the questions below.)

1. Identify the assessments you will perform when Mr. J. is initially admitted and your rationale for each.

After several doses of Vasodilan, you check Mr. J.'s vital signs and find that his pulse is 98 and BP 80/60. He is complaining of dizziness and has palpable peripheral pulses.

2. Identify and prioritize your nursing actions.

Mr. J.'s physician changes his medication to pentoxifylline (Trental).

3. Discuss the discharge teaching you will do with Mr. J.

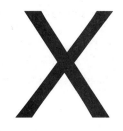

DRUGS AFFECTING THE DIGESTIVE SYSTEM

59

Physiology of the Digestive System

Digestive System Diagram

Match the organ with its function by filling in the blanks in Figure 59-1 with the letters below.

A. Absorption of most oral medications takes place here.

B. Water is absorbed here.

C. Secretes enzymes necessary for digestion.

D. Most drugs are metabolized here.

E. Releases bile when fats are present in the intestine.

F. Starch digestion starts here.

G. Protein breakdown occurs here.

Figure 59-1

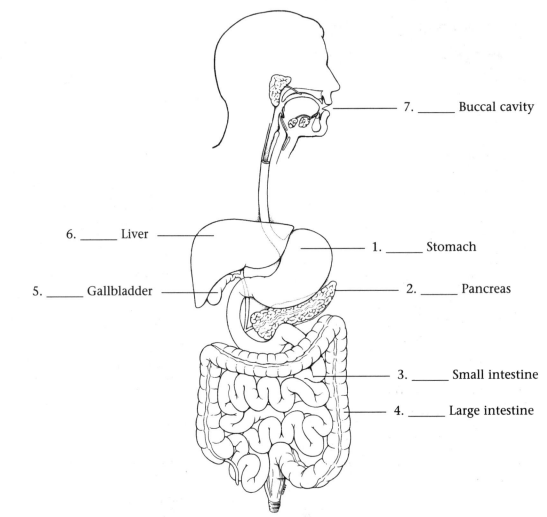

7. _____ Buccal cavity

6. _____ Liver

1. _____ Stomach

5. _____ Gallbladder

2. _____ Pancreas

3. _____ Small intestine

4. _____ Large intestine

REVIEW QUESTIONS

1. When liver function is impaired, this substance can accumulate
   a. fat-soluble vitamins.
   b. hormones.
   c. glucose.
   d. cholesterol.

2. Gastric juice has a pH of
   a. 1–3.
   b. 4–5.
   c. 6–7.
   d. 8 or above.

3. The major digestive enzyme in gastric juice is
    a. enterogastrone.
    b. gastrin.
    c. pepsin.
    d. lipase.

4. Bile is secreted by the
    a. gallbladder.
    b. liver.
    c. pancreas.
    d. small intestine.

5. The pancreas secretes all of the following, except:
    a. Amylase.
    b. Lipase.
    c. Cholesterol.
    d. Trypsin.

6. The stomach empties in about
    a. 1 hour.
    b. 2 hours.
    c. 3 hours.
    d. 4 hours.

7. For the most part, digestion and absorption occur in the
    a. stomach.
    b. small intestine.
    c. large intestine.
    d. liver.

8. The liver breaks down worn out erythrocytes and forms this waste product, which is excreted in bile.
    a. Bile salts.
    b. Bilirubin.
    c. Cholesterol.
    d. Fatty acids.

9. The body organ that produces 20% of the total body heat is the
    a. gallbladder.
    b. pancreas.
    c. liver.
    d. large intestine.

10. Blood flow to the GI tract increases with
    a. temperature extremes.
    b. pain.
    c. strenuous exercise.
    d. digestion.

60

Drugs Used in Peptic Ulcer Disease

MATCHING EXERCISE

Terms and Concepts

Match the concept with the term for it.

1. _____ Prevent the release of gastric acid into the stomach lumen.

2. _____ Inhibit gastric acid secretion.

3. _____ Increase mucus production.

4. _____ Used with other agents to further reduce gastric acid secretion.

5. _____ React with hydrochloric acid in the stomach to raise the pH (alkaline).

6. _____ Large doses are required, cause constipation; the client may develop hypophosphatemia.

7. _____ Have a high neutralizing capacity, cause diarrhea and hypermagnesemia.

8. _____ Rapid onset of action, may cause alkalosis.

9. _____ Aluminum-based antacid used to lower serum phosphate levels.

10. _____ An antiflatulent.

A. Anticholinergic agents.

B. Gastric acid pump inhibitors.

C. Histamine-2 receptor blocking agents.

D. Prostaglandins.

E. Antacids.

F. Calcium compounds.

G. Amphogel.

H. Sodium bicarbonate.

I. Magnesium compounds.

J. Simethicone (Mylicon).

TRUE OR FALSE

1. _____ Alcohol and caffeine can cause gastric irritation.

2. _____ Protein and calcium in milk decrease secretion of gastric acid.

3. _____ Ulcers are usually treated with sucralfate (Carafate) for 2–4 weeks.

4. _____ Antacids increase the effectiveness of cimetidine (Tagamet) and sucralfate (Carafate).

5. _____ Avoiding highly spiced and gas-forming foods prevents ulcer formation.

6. _____ Stress stimulates gastric acid secretion.

7. _____ Omeprazole should be swallowed whole.

8. _____ Magnesium-containing antacids cause constipation.

9. _____ Proton pump inhibitors prevent the release of gastric acid.

10. _____ H_2 receptor blockers decrease the acidity of the gastric juice.

FILL IN THE BLANKS

Complete the following sentences.

1. Besides peptic ulcer disease, antacids are also used in the treatment of _____, _____, and _____.

2. Omeprazole (Prilosec) inhibits gastric acid secretion by preventing the release of _____ into the stomach lumen.

3. Cimetidine (Tagamet) decreases the _____ and _____ of gastric juices.

4. Ranitidine (Zantac) is more _____ than cimetidine (Tagamet) and has fewer _____.

5. Famotidine (_____) and nizatidine (_____) are also used to treat ulcers but are less likely to cause _____ and _____.

6. Misoprostol (_____) is indicated for clients with a high risk of _____.

7. Sucralfate (_____) adheres to the _____ and forms a protective _____ to promote _____.

8. Risk factors for peptic ulcer disease include

   a. _____

   b. _____

   c. _____

   d. _____

   e. _____

   f. _____

MATCHING EXERCISE

The drugs below interact with cimetidine (Tagamet). Match them with their classification.

1. _____ Antiarrhythmics.

2. _____ Anticoagulant.

3. _____ Benzodiazepine antianxiety or hypnotic agents.

4. _____ Beta-adrenergic blocking agents.

5. _____ Bronchodilator.

6. _____ Calcium channel blocker.

7. _____ Tricyclic antidepressant.

8. _____ Anticonvulsants.

A. Carbamazepine, phenytoin.

B. Verapamil.

C. Alprazolam, chlordiazepoxide, diazepam, flurazepam, triazolam.

D. Lidocaine, quinidine.

E. Theophylline.

F. Warfarin.

G. Labetalol, metoprolol, propranolol.

H. Amitriptyline.

CROSSWORD PUZZLE

Across

1. A synthetic form of prostaglandin E; helpful to counter gastric irritation caused by NSAIDs.

4. Antacids with high _____ content are contraindicated in edematous states.

9. _____ carbonate overuse may cause hypercalcemia.

10. Calcium antacids are rarely used for peptic ulcers because they cause _____ of gastric acid.

Down

2. This type of drug can cause abortion.

3. It is important that a patient be matched with an antacid that has this quality.

5. A drug that can prevent the development of stress ulcers.

6. Antacids containing this element may cause constipation.

7. A gastric acid-inhibiting drug in a time-release capsule.

8. A cytoprotective drug that binds to ulcerated mucosa.

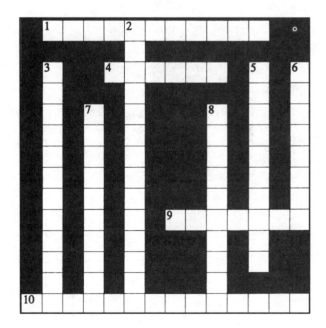

REVIEW QUESTIONS

1. The ideal time to take antacids is
   a. 2 hours after meals.
   b. 1 hour before or after other drugs.
   c. ½ hour before meals with milk.
   d. with meals.

2. Your client is taking cimetidine (Tagamet). Which of the following statements would lead you to believe that he has understood the instructions?
   a. "I will take an antacid an hour before meals with the cimetidine (Tagamet)."
   b. "I will chew the tablets before swallowing them."
   c. "I will take cimetidine (Tagamet) with meals."
   d. "I will always take cimetidine with orange juice because it will enhance the absorption of the cimetidine."

3. Mr. J. has been treated for peptic ulcer disease with sucralfate (Carafate). His physician has recently added cimetidine (Tagamet). What adverse effect should you be observing for?
   a. abdominal pain.
   b. nausea and vomiting.
   c. constipation.
   d. blurred vision.

4. Which of the following medications is effective in preventing GI bleeding when administered with NSAIDs (nonsteroidal antiinflammatory drugs)?
   a. Famotidine (Pepcid).
   b. Nizatidine (Axid).
   c. Misoprostol (Cytotec).
   d. Sucralfate (Carafate).

5. The physician orders ranitidine (Zantac) 50 mg in 100 cc D5W to be infused over 30 minutes. How fast will you run the IV (using macro gtt tubing, 1 cc = 10 gtt)?
   a. 27 gtt/minute.
   b. 33 gtt/minute.
   c. 42 gtt/minute.
   d. 50 gtt/minute.

6. Mrs. H., a 79-year-old female with peptic ulcer disease, is taking cimetidine (Tagamet). When you enter her room, you find that she is confused. You should
   a. hold the medication until you have gotten her out of bed.
   b. hold the medication and contact her physician.
   c. stop the medication.
   d. administer the medication as ordered.

7. Persons taking aluminum compounds to neutralize stomach acid should be assessed for
   a. constipation.
   b. hyperphosphatemia.
   c. hypomagnesemia.
   d. diarrhea.

8. Mrs. H. is having a great deal of flatulence after her surgery. Which of the following antacids would be most helpful to her?
   a. Maalox.
   b. Gelusil.
   c. Titralac.
   d. Aludrox.

9. Magnesium-based antacids are contraindicated in
   a. hypertension.
   b. congestive heart failure.
   c. hepatic failure.
   d. renal failure.

10. Mrs. H. is in chronic end-stage renal failure. The physician prescribes Amphojel for her, to
    a. decrease her absorption of phosphates.
    b. increase her serum calcium.
    c. prevent gastric irritation.
    d. prevent constipation.

CRITICAL THINKING CASE STUDY

Mr. J. is admitted with a duodenal ulcer because he is actively bleeding. The physician starts him on cimetidine (Tagamet).

1. Identify why Tagamet is ordered for Mr. J.

2. If 300 mg of Tagamet in 100 ml of D5W is to infuse over 20 minutes using macrodrip tubing (10 gtt = 1 ml), at how many drops per minute will you run the IV?

3. Identify the adverse reactions of the Tagamet you will be observing for.

Mr. J. is no longer bleeding and the physician starts him on sucralfate (Carafate).

4. Identify what you will be observing for.

5. Identify what foods should be avoided in peptic ulcer disease and explain why.

6. Discuss the instructions you will give Mr. J. before discharge.

61

Laxatives and Cathartics

MATCHING EXERCISE

Terms and Concepts

Match the concept with the term for it.

1. _____ These substances swell and become gel-like and stimulate peristalsis and defecation.

2. _____ This laxative is also used to treat hepatic encephalopathy.

3. _____ These substances increase osmotic pressure in the intestinal lumen, causing water to be retained.

4. _____ These drugs irritate the GI mucosa, pulling water into the bowel lumen.

5. _____ Used as a suppository, it stimulates bowel evacuation by irritating the rectal mucosa.

6. _____ This lubricates the intestine by retarding colonic absorption of fecal water.

7. _____ A laxative that decreases the production of ammonia in the intestine.

8. _____ A substance commonly mixed with Kayexalate to prevent constipation.

9. _____ Used for fecal impaction.

10. _____ An adverse effect of the administration of mineral oil.

11. _____ Saline cathartics are contraindicated in renal disease because they may cause this.

12. _____ A product used to cleanse the bowel before surgery.

13. _____ This saline cathartic is less likely to produce hyponatremia because it has sodium sulfate as its major component.

14. _____ This laxative should be taken with a full glass of water.

15. _____ Discoloration of urine may occur with this laxative.

A. Saline cathartics.

B. Mineral oil.

C. Sorbitol.

D. Stimulant cathartics.

E. Lactulose.

F. Bulk-forming laxatives.

G. Glycerin.

H. Lactulose (Chronulac).

I. Oil retention enema.

J. Decreased absorption of fat-soluble vitamins.

K. Anemia.

L. Hypermagnesemia.

M. Hyponatremia.

N. Magnesium citrate.

O. Polyethylene glycol–electrolyte solution (GoLytely).

P. Cascara sagrada.

Q. Psyllium preparations (Metamucil).

DEFINITIONS

Define the following terms.

1. Surfactant laxatives

_____

2. Defecation

_____

REVIEW QUESTIONS

1. Which of the following statements by Mrs. H. leads you to believe that she has understood how to use Metamucil?

   a. "I will drink the Metamucil as soon as I have it mixed."

   b. "I will mix the dry medication with applesauce."

   c. "I will use milk of magnesia in conjunction with this medication until I am having daily bowel movements."

   d. "I will decrease the roughage in my diet while I am using this medication."

2. A laxative used with Kayexalate to prevent constipation and aid in expulsion of the Kayexalate.

   a. Docusate sodium (Colace).

   b. Polyethylene glycol–electrolyte solution (GoLytely).

   c. Lactulose (Chronulac).

   d. Sorbitol.

3. Mr. J. is to receive polyethylene glycol–electrolyte solution (GoLytely) for bowel cleansing before an endoscopic procedure. Which instructions should you give Mr. J.?

   a. "Take 1 gram every 4 hours followed by 8 ounces of fluid."

   b. "Take 1 ounce every hour until midnight."

   c. "Take 8 ounces every 10 minutes until the 4 liters are gone."

   d. "Take 1 ounce at bedtime and you will receive a cleansing enema in the morning."

4. An adverse effect of the administration of bulk-forming laxatives is

   a. impaction.

   b. vomiting.

   c. diarrhea.

   d. lower GI bleeding.

5. Administration of mineral oil can decrease the absorption of fat-soluble vitamins if continued for longer than

   a. 1 week.

   b. 2 weeks.

   c. 2 months.

   d. 6 months.

6. Long-term use of saline cathartics can produce this electrolyte imbalance.

   a. Hypermagnesemia.

   b. Hypokalemia.

   c. Hypochloremia.

   d. Hyperphosphatemia.

7. Medications that increase the effectiveness of laxatives when administered with them are

   a. anticholinergics.

   b. beta-adrenergic blockers.

   c. cholinergics.

   d. diuretics.

8. Before taking laxatives for constipation, Mrs. C. should

   a. drink 2000–3000 cc of fluid for several days.

   b. go to the bathroom every 2 hours.

   c. eat foods high in potassium.

   d. take a cleansing enema.

9. Mr. J. has recently suffered a myocardial infarction. Which of the following would be the most effective in preventing straining?

   a. Docusate sodium (Colace).

   b. Polyethylene glycol–electrolyte solution (GoLytely).

   c. Lactulose (Chronulac).

   d. Sorbitol.

10. Which of the following laxatives acts by increasing osmotic pressure in the intestinal lumen and causing water to be retained?

    a. Lubricant laxatives.

    b. Bulk-forming laxatives.

    c. Magnesium citrate.

    d. Stimulant cathartics.

CRITICAL THINKING CASE STUDY

Mrs. J., a 79-year-old female, has recently been admitted to your nursing home. She has had a problem with constipation for a number of years and is a chronic laxative user.

1. Identify nonmedicinal ways of dealing with constipation.

Two days later, Mrs. J. still has not had a bowel movement. You contact the physician and he asks you what you think would work best for Mrs. J.

2. Identify your response and the rationale for your response.

62

Antidiarrheals

TRUE OR FALSE

1. _____ Very hot foods can cause diarrhea.

2. _____ Persons with a deficiency of lactase may have diarrhea when they eat dairy products.

3. _____ Severe diarrhea can result in metabolic acidosis.

4. _____ Diarrhea can be a symptom of stress in certain individuals.

5. _____ Hypothyroidism increases bowel motility.

6. _____ Chronic diarrhea can result in malnutrition and anemia.

7. _____ Psyllium preparations (Metamucil) are useful for both diarrhea and constipation.

8. _____ Withholding fluids is an effective way of treating diarrhea.

9. _____ Intestinal tumors can cause diarrhea.

10. _____ The drug of choice for treating diarrhea resulting from chronic inflammatory bowel disease is diphenoxylate with atropine sulfate (Lomotil).

11. _____ Cholestyramine (Questran) is the drug of choice for treating diarrhea due to bile salts.

12. _____ Loperamide (Imodium) is contraindicated for treating diarrhea due to bile salts.

13. _____ Side effects of diphenoxylate (Lomotil) include bradycardia and elevated blood sugar.

14. _____ Alcohol will decrease the effect of antidiarrheal drugs.

15. _____ You should report to a physician if your diarrhea persists for more than 3 days.

FILL IN THE BLANKS

Complete the following sentences.

1. Causes of diarrhea include

   a. _____

   b. _____

   c. _____

   d. _____

   e. _____

   f. _____

2. Nonmedicinal approaches to diarrhea treatment include

   a. _____

   ‘b. _____

   c. _____

   d. _____

REVIEW QUESTIONS

1. Which of the following medications is used to treat the diarrhea associated with pseudomembranous colitis?

   a. Lactobacillus.

   b. Vancomycin (Vancocin).

   c. Pepto-Bismol.

   d. Psyllium preparations (Metamucil).

2. Cholestyramine (Questran) is most effective in treating the diarrhea associated with

   a. Crohn's disease.

   b. Bile salts.

   c. Salmonella.

   d. Bacillary dysentery.

3. Which of the following medications, if administered with diphenoxylate with atropine sulfate (Lomotil) will increase its antidiarrheal effects?

   a. Antihistamines.

   b. Cholinergic agents.

   c. Thiazide diuretics.

   d. Beta-adrenergic blockers.

4. Which of the following statements by Mr. B. leads you to believe that he has understood the teaching you have done regarding loperamide (Imodium)?

    a. "It is not uncommon for there to be an increase in diarrhea initially."

    b. "I may experience dry mouth and urinary retention from this medication."

    c. "I should take the medication with foods high in potassium."

    d. "If I have a weight loss of more than 2 lb I will contact my physician."

5. The nurse should assess for which of the following adverse reactions when administering colestipol (Colestid)?

    a. Nausea and vomiting.

    b. Hypertension.

    c. Constipation.

    d. A papular rash.

6. Which of the following antidiarrheal medications is used to treat diarrhea associated with ulcerative colitis?

    a. Cholestyramine (Questran).

    b. Psyllium preparations (Metamucil).

    c. Loperamide (Imodium).

    d. Sulfasalazine (Azulfidine).

7. Your neighbor calls you because she has been having diarrhea for 2 days. What advice should you give her?

    a. Drink 2–3 liters of water every day.

    b. Restrict your oral intake to decrease bowel stimulation.

    c. Drink plenty of fluids that contain calories and electrolytes.

    d. Eat dry crackers and cereal and only take sips of water.

8. Which of the following instructions should you give to your client who is taking cholestyramine (Questran) for diarrhea?

    a. "Always take the medication on an empty stomach."

    b. "Add at least 30 cc of water to each dose."

    c. "Do not take the medication within 4 hours of other medications."

    d. "If the medication does not control the diarrhea in 2 weeks, contact your physician."

9. Mr. J. has a history of diabetes mellitus, COPD, glaucoma, and hypothyroidism. For which of these disorders would the use of diphenoxylate with atropine sulfate (Lomotil) be contraindicated?

    a. Hypothyroidism.

    b. Glaucoma.

    c. COPD.

    d. Diabetes mellitus.

10. M.J., age 4, is admitted with an overdose of loperamide (Imodium). Which medication listed below is the antidote for Imodium?

    a. Lactulose (Chronulac).

    b. Diphenhydramine hydrochloride (Benadryl).

    c. Epinephrine.

    d. Naloxone (Narcan).

CRITICAL THINKING CASE STUDY

You are a hospice nurse caring for Mr. N. who has an inoperable cancerous intestinal tumor and is receiving Sandostatin to help control his daily diarrhea. (The learner may need to use additional sources to answer the questions below.)

1. Identify the instructions you will give Mr. N.

The physician also orders Metamucil.

2. Specify the rationale for this order.

3. Identify the nursing assessments that you will make during each visit.

Mr. N. continues to have diarrhea and is having a significant amount of abdominal pain. His physician orders 2 mg of morphine q2h.

4. Identify how this will help Mr. N.'s diarrhea.

63

Antiemetics

MATCHING EXERCISE

Terms and Concepts

Match the concept with the term for it.

1. _____ A benzodiazepine useful in treating persons who experience anticipatory nausea and vomiting.

2. _____ A corticosteroid used for treatment of nausea and vomiting.

3. _____ An anticholinergic drug effective in treating motion sickness.

4. _____ Administered 30 minutes before cisplatin to prevent/minimize nausea and vomiting.

5. _____ Administered orally at 15-minute intervals until vomiting stops.

6. _____ Used during surgical procedures to prevent nausea and vomiting.

7. _____ These drugs block the action of acetylcholine in the brain.

8. _____ These drugs block dopamine from receptor sites in the brain.

9. _____ The vomiting center is located here.

10. _____ Along with hydroxyzine (Vistaril), one of the most commonly used antiemetic agents.

11. _____ A phenothiazine that acts on the CTZ and vomiting center.

12. _____ A cannabinoid used to manage nausea and vomiting during cancer treatment.

13. _____ An adverse effect of antiemetics.

14. _____ Vestibular branch of auditory nerve.

15. _____ Cerebral cortex, vestibular apparatus of the ear, and neurons in the fourth ventricle.

A. Dexamethasone (Decadron).

B. Metoclopramide (Reglan).

C. Phosphorated carbohydrate solution (Emetrol).

D. Antihistamines.

E. Medulla oblongata.

F. Promethazine (Phenergan).

G. Phenothiazines.

H. Droperidol (Inapsine).

I. Scopolamine (Transderm Scop).

J. Lorazepam (Ativan).

K. Cerebrum.

L. Dronabinol (Marinol).

M. Concerned with equilibrium.

N. Drowsiness.

O. Prochlorperazine (Compazine).

P. Chemoreceptor trigger zone.

REVIEW QUESTIONS

1. The following medications, if administered concurrently with antiemetic agents, will increase their effects.

   a. Anticholinergic agents.

   b. Thiazide diuretics.

   c. Cholinergic agents.

   d. Calcium channel blockers.

2. The physician orders ondanestron (Zofran) for the management of Mrs. G.'s nausea and vomiting associated with her chemotherapy. Two days after starting the medication you find that Mrs. G. has a pulse rate of 108, a BP of 90/40, a macular rash, and a headache. Which of these symptoms may be related to the use of nabilone (Cesamet)?

   a. Tachycardia.

   b. Hypotension.

   c. Rash.

   d. Headache.

3. Persons using antiemetics may experience anticholinergic effects, which include

   a. dysphoria, drowsiness, and dizziness.

   b. dyskinesia, dystonia, and akathisia.

   c. dry mouth, blurred vision, and urinary retention.

   d. hypotension, confusion, and shuffling gait.

4. Which of the following statements by your client leads you to believe that she has understood the teaching you have done regarding prochlorperazine (Compazine)?

   a. "During episodes of nausea, I will drink clear liquids."

   b. "If I vomit, this medication can be administered rectally."

   c. "This medication should be taken on a full stomach."

   d. "I will need to decrease my sodium intake while I am on this medication."

5. The use of promethazine (Phenergan) is contraindicated in

   a. children under the age of 12 years.

   b. preoperative patients.

   c. pregnant women.

   d. persons under 100 lb.

6. Which of the following antiemetics is commonly used preoperatively with meperidine (Demerol) and atropine?

   a. Promethazine (Phenergan).

   b. Prochlorperazine (Compazine).

   c. Diphenhydramine (Benadryl).

   d. Scopolamine.

7. Which of the following statements by your client leads you to believe that she needs additional instruction regarding antiemetics?

   a. "I will not drive while I am taking this medication."

   b. "Before I use any other medications I will contact my physician."

   c. "If I become drowsy I will stop taking the medication."

   d. "If I experience adverse reactions to this medication, I will contact my physician."

8. Mrs. P. becomes nauseated the night before her chemotherapy treatments. Her physician believes that she is experiencing anticipatory nausea. Which of the following medications would be most effective for Mrs. P.'s nausea?

   a. Lorazepam (Ativan).

   b. Diphenhydramine (Benadryl).

   c. Hydroxyzine (Atarax).

   d. Trimethobenzamide (Tigan).

9. Mr. J. is going on an ocean cruise and is concerned about nausea and vomiting. His physician orders a scopolamine (Transderm Scop) patch. Which statement by Mr. J. leads you to believe that he understands how to use the patch?

   a. "I will put it on in the morning and take it off at night."

   b. "I will place the patch behind my ear and replace it every 3 days."

   c. "I will only use the patch if I feel nauseated or begin to vomit."

   d. "I will apply a thin layer of powder before I apply the patch to prevent irritation."

10. Mr. S. is receiving a phenothiazine for severe nausea. The nurse needs to assess Mr. S. for adverse effects, which include

    a. increased urinary output.

    b. hypotension and drowsiness.

    c. dizziness and depression.

    d. anorexia.

CRITICAL THINKING CASE STUDY

After radiation therapy, Mrs. B., who has a 10-year history of hypertension, experiences nausea and vomiting. Her physician orders lorazepam (Ativan).

1. Discuss why this medication was ordered.

2. Identify other measures that may be helpful in controlling nausea and vomiting.

Mrs. B.'s nausea and vomiting continue, so her physician adds prochlorperazine (Compazine).

3. Explain why this drug was chosen and the expected outcome after the drug is administered.

XI

DRUGS USED IN SPECIAL CONDITIONS

64

Antineoplastic Drugs

MATCHING EXERCISE

Terms and Concepts

Match the antineoplastic agent with the disease process it is used for.

1. _____ Chronic granulocytic leukemia.

2. _____ Hodgkin's disease.

3. _____ Multiple myeloma.

4. _____ To prevent the rejection of renal transplants.

5. _____ Acute lymphoblastic leukemia in children.

6. _____ Carcinoma of the breast.

7. _____ Kaposi's sarcoma.

8. _____ Advanced prostatic cancer.

9. _____ Advanced endometrial carcinoma.

10. _____ Rhabdomyosarcoma, Wilms' tumor.

11. _____ Squamous cell carcinoma.

12. _____ Palliation of ovarian cancer.

13. _____ Cancer of the testes, bladder, ovaries.

14. _____ Advanced breast cancer in post-menopausal women.

15. _____ Used as an adjunct for palliation of symptoms in acute leukemia, Hodgkin's disease.

A. Melphalan (Alkeran).

B. Methotrexate (Mexate).

C. Medroxyprogesterone (Depo-Provera).

D. Busulfan (Myleran).

E. Dactinomycin (Cosmegen).

F. Goserelin (Zoladex).

G. Daunorubicin (Cerubidin).

H. Fluorouracil (5-FU) (Adrucil).

I. Azathioprine (Imuran).

J. Cyclophosphamide (Cytoxan).

K. Carboplatin (Paraplatin).

L. Bleomycin (Blenoxane).

M. Tamoxifen (Nolvadex).

N. Prednisone (Meticorten).

O. Cisplatin (Platinol).

TRUE OR FALSE

1. _____ A cancer develops from a single normal cell that is transformed into a malignant cell.

2. _____ Viruses have been linked to the development of certain types of cancers.

3. _____ The incidence of cancer of the stomach is higher in the USA than in Japan.

4. _____ Lung cancer is the leading cause of cancer death in both men and women.

5. _____ Cancers of the mouth, throat, and esophagus are associated with excessive use of alcohol.

6. _____ A diet high in fat has been linked to breast cancer.

7. _____ Multiple myeloma is derived from epithelial tissue and is the most common type of malignant tumor.

8. _____ Some antineoplastic drugs are cell-cycle specific and need to be administered continuously.

9. _____ Alkylating agents such as nitrogen mustard act during the dividing and resting stages of the cell cycle.

10. _____ Alkaloids are derived from plants.

11. _____ A blood test for carcinoembryonic antigen (CEA) is an accurate blood test commonly used for the diagnosis of cancer.

12. _____ Alopecia is a common side effect of several antineoplastic medications.

13. _____ The rapid breakdown or destruction of malignant cells can result in hypercalcemia.

14. _____ If extravasation of a chemotherapeutic agent occurs, the nurse should apply warm compresses and elevate the extremity.

15. _____ Antineoplastic drugs can exert adverse effects on nurses who prepare and administer them.

FILL IN THE BLANKS

Cell Cycle

In the spaces provided in Figure 64-1, explain what happens during each phase of cell replication.

Figure 64-1

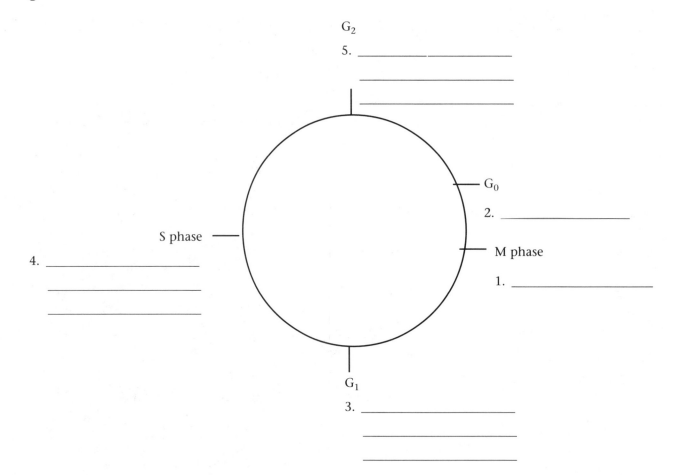

REVIEW QUESTIONS

1. Your client has been started on carmustine (BiCNU) for malignant myeloma. Which of the following statements by your client leads you to believe that he has understood the teaching you have done?

   a. "If I have a fever or notice unusual bruising, I will call my doctor."

   b. "If I get short of breath, I will just rest."

   c. "Blood in the urine is common so I won't be concerned."

   d. "I will call the doctor if I am nauseated."

2. Your client expresses concern that she will lose her hair during chemotherapy. Identify your best response.

   a. "Hair loss is temporary and reversible when the drug is stopped."

   b. "You may not lose your hair. Just wait and see what happens."

   c. "If you get a permanent wave, the hair that you have will appear thicker."

   d. "Some people lose their hair, but it grows back in nice and thick so don't worry."

3. Alkaloid agents are more effective

   a. against resting cells.

   b. when there is organ impairment.

   c. when cancerous cells have metastasized.

   d. against dividing cells.

4. An example of a hormone inhibitor used to treat breast cancer is

   a. ethinyl estradiol (Estinyl).

   b. medroxyprogesterone (Depo-Provera).

   c. tamoxifen (Nolvadex).

   d. cisplatin (Platinol).

5. You know that your teaching has been effective with a client receiving vincristine (Oncovin) if he states

   a. "I will avoid foods high in roughage."

   b. "I will drink plenty of fluids."

   c. "I will avoid foods that are high in iron."

   d. "I will weigh myself daily."

6. Acute lymphocytic leukemia is treated with methotrexate (Mexate) to

   a. decrease overproduction of abnormal red blood cells.

   b. decrease platelet production.

   c. decrease production of lymphocytes.

   d. decrease overproduction of abnormal white blood cells.

7. Which of the following drugs, if administered with methotrexate (Mexate), will increase its effect?

   a. Phenytoin (Dilantin).

   b. Furosemide (Lasix).

   c. Propranolol (Inderal).

   d. Verapamil (Calan).

8. When administering daunorubicin (Cerubidin) to Mr. H., the nurse should assess him for:

   a. cardiotoxicity.

   b. pulmonary toxicity.

   c. neurotoxicity.

   d. renal toxicity.

9. Which of these instructions should you give Mr. C., who has advanced prostatic cancer with bone metastasis and is to receive goserelin (Zoladex)?

   a. "You may experience hot flashes and nausea and vomiting."

   b. "This medication may cause breast enlargement and hair loss."

   c. "Your symptoms may worsen during the first few days of treatment, especially your bone pain."

   d. "This medication can cause fever, dyspnea, nausea, vomiting, and diarrhea."

10. Alopecia is a common adverse effect associated with which of the following medications?

    a. Diethylstilbestrol (Stilbestrol).

    b. Megestrol (Megace).

    c. Medroxyprogesterone (Depo-Provera).

    d. Doxorubicin (Adriamycin).

CRITICAL THINKING CASE STUDY

Mrs. J. is receiving a combination chemotherapy regimen (FAC) of 5-fluorouracil, doxorubicin (Adriamycin), and cyclophosphamide (Cytoxan) for breast cancer.

1. Discuss with Mrs. J. why this regimen was chosen and what she can expect.

Mrs. J. begins to lose her hair, has developed stomatitis, and is extremely depressed.

2. Describe your nursing intervention.

Mrs. J. calls you to come quickly because there is blood in her urine. You examine the urine and find that it is red.

3. Discuss what your nursing actions will be.

One week after the initial treatment you find that Mrs. J. has a respiratory rate of 28 and a pulse of 102 and rales are audible in her lung bases bilaterally.

4. Describe what you will do.

65

Drugs Used in Ophthalmic Conditions

MATCHING EXERCISES

Terms and Concepts

Match the concept with the term for it.

1. _____ May follow topical steroid therapy or injury.
2. _____ May be caused by inadequate lacrimation.
3. _____ A chronic infection in the lash follicles on the eyelid.
4. _____ Characterized by redness and watery discharge.
5. _____ Increased intraocular pressure.
6. _____ White, opaque, fibrous tissue that covers $5/6$ of eyeball.
7. _____ The innermost layer of the eyeball.
8. _____ Constriction of the pupil.
9. _____ Dilation of the pupil.
10. _____ An elastic transparent structure that focuses light rays to form images on the retina.

A. Glaucoma.
B. Conjunctivitis.
C. Blepharitis.
D. Keratitis.
E. Corneal ulcer.
F. Retina.
G. Miosis.
H. Lens.
I. Mydriasis.
J. Sclera.
K. Cornea.

FILL IN THE BLANKS

Complete the following sentences.

1. Autonomic drugs are used preoperatively to _____.

2. Corticosteroids such as dexamethasone (Decadron Phosphate) are used to treat _____ of the eye.

3. A carbonic anhydrase inhibitor such as acetazolamide (Diamox) _____ intraocular pressure.

4. Fluorescein is a _____ used to _____ lesions or foreign bodies in the eye.

5. Cholinergic drugs used for _____ are instilled in the eye _____ times per day and cause the pupil to _____.

6. Anticholinergic drugs such as atropine are used before eye exams to _____ the pupil. Their use is usually contraindicated in the presence of _____.

7. Ocusert is replaced _____ and is used for long-term treatment of _____.

8. Emergency treatment for chemical burns of the eyes includes _____

9. The drug therapy for eye infections caused by the herpes simplex virus is _____ (_____).

NAME THAT DRUG

Identify the medications that cause the following adverse effects.

1. _____ Dehydration and hyperglycemia.

2. _____ Bradycardia and bronchoconstriction.

3. _____ Dry mouth and tachycardia.

4. _____ Nausea and paresthesias.

5. _____ Hypertension and arrhythmias.

DRUG CLASSIFICATION

Give an example of one drug in each classification and specify what it is used for.

	Medication	Use
1. Adrenergic		
2. Anti-adrenergic		
3. Cholinergic		
4. Anticholinesterase		
5. Anticholinergic		
6. Carbonic anhydrase inhibitor		
7. Osmotic agents		
8. Alpha$_2$ adrenergic agonist		
9. Anesthetics		
10. Antiseptic		
11. Lubricants		
12. Prostaglandin		

REVIEW QUESTIONS

1. When administering eyedrops, you should
   a. not remove crusts around the eye before administering the medication.
   b. pull the lower lid down, drop the medication in the eye, and do not touch the eye with the applicator.
   c. pull the upper lid up and have the person look down; do not have them close their eyes for 1 minute after you have put the drops in.
   d. place one drop in each eye, wait 5 minutes, then place a second drop.

2. Your client is to go home on polyvinyl alcohol (Liquifilm). Your instructions should include the following:
   a. "Use one or two drops as often as you feel you need to."
   b. "Nausea, vomiting, and diarrhea are common side effects."
   c. "Lie down for 5 minutes after taking the medications."
   d. "If you experience blurred vision and photophobia, contact your physician."

3. Dipivefrin (Propine), an adrenergic drug, reduces intraocular pressure by
   a. contracting the sphincter muscle of the eye.
   b. preventing ciliary muscle spasm.
   c. decreasing production of aqueous humor.
   d. increasing outflow of aqueous humor.

4. Clients receiving demecarium bromide (Humorsol) will experience
   a. miosis.
   b. mydriasis.
   c. no pupillary change.
   d. double vision.

5. A person receiving anticholinesterase agents for a long period of time might experience side effects, including
   a. dehydration and hyperglycemia.
   b. corneal ulcerations.
   c. cataract formation.
   d. hypertension and dysrhythmias.

6. Which of these statements demonstrates that the client understands the teaching you have done about pilocarpine (Pilocar)?
   a. "This drug can cause irritation and discomfort. My eyes may be red after I use these drops."
   b. "I know that I will have dry eyes so I will use a lubricant after the pilocarpine."
   c. "The dosage of pilocarpine will need to be increased as I get older."
   d. "I can no longer drive an automobile."

7. Osmotic agents are used for
   a. treatment of chronic glaucoma.
   b. preoperative treatment for intraocular surgery.
   c. treatment of conjunctivitis.
   d. reduction of adhesion formation with uveitis.

8. The drug of choice for treating eye infections caused by herpes simplex virus is
   a. neomycin.
   b. trifluridine (Viroptic).
   c. sulfapred.
   d. natamycin (Natacyn).

9. Silver nitrate is used in newborns to prevent eye damage from
   a. Trichomonas.
   b. Candida albicans.
   c. staphylococcal infections.
   d. gonorrhea.

10. Medications that could elevate intraocular pressure include
    a. ibuprofen (Advil).
    b. meperidine (Demerol).
    c. prochlorperazine (Compazine).
    d. dexamethasone (Decadron).

CRITICAL THINKING CASE STUDY

Mrs. R. has come to the office for an eye exam because she had difficulty threading a needle. Her intraocular pressure is significantly elevated so her physician orders timolol maleate (Timoptic) and pilocarpine (Pilocar).

1. Discuss why these medications were ordered for Mrs. R.

2. Identify the instructions that you will give Mrs. R.

Mrs. R. complains of burning when she instills the drops and asks you how long she will have to continue using them.

3. Discuss how you will respond to Mrs. R.

Mrs. R.'s brother also has glaucoma and she is concerned about her children.

4. Discuss how you will respond to Mrs. R.

66

Drugs Used in Dermatologic Conditions

MATCHING EXERCISE

Terms and Concepts

Match the concept with the term for it.

1. _____ Pigment producing cells.

2. _____ An inflammatory response of the skin to various injuries.

3. _____ "Hives."

4. _____ Chronic skin disorder characterized by dry scaling lesions.

5. _____ Characterized by erythema, tenderness, and edema.

6. _____ An infection of the hair follicles.

7. _____ "Boils."

8. _____ A contagious skin infection.

9. _____ This fungal infection can occur following the use of broad spectrum antibiotics.

10. _____ "Athlete's foot."

11. _____ A viral infection of the skin.

12. _____ Follicles become infected and pustules, cysts, and abscesses are formed.

13. _____ A drying agent used for exudative lesions.

14. _____ An agent used to debride wounds.

15. _____ An agent used to remove warts.

16. _____ An oil-based substance useful in chronic skin conditions characterized by dry lesions.

17. _____ These substances may be used on the face or hairy moist areas.

18. _____ Suspensions of insoluble substances that cool, dry, and protect the skin.

19. _____ A substance that absorbs, cools, and protects.

20. _____ A semi-solid preparation that adheres strongly to the area of application.

A. Dermatitis.

B. Psoriasis.

C. Folliculitis.

D. Impetigo.

E. Tinea pedis.

F. Warts.

G. Astringent.

H. Enzyme.

I. Acne vulgaris.

J. Oral candidiasis.

K. Furuncles.

L. Cellulitis.

M. Urticaria.

N. Melanocytes.

O. Keratolytic agent.

P. Creams.

Q. Powders.

R. Paste.

S. Lotion.

T. Ointment.

REVIEW QUESTIONS

1. Mrs. J. has an infected leg wound and the physician has ordered modified Dakin's solution. Mrs. J. asks you why her physician ordered this. The best reply would be

   a. "This solution exerts bactericidal action by releasing hydrochloric acid."

   b. "This is an excellent cleaning agent. It will dissolve necrotic materials."

   c. "Drug resistance can develop from oral agents; topical steroids are better."

   d. "When the skin is broken, more of the drug is absorbed systemically, so this solution is more effective than oral agents."

2. An effective topical agent for psoriasis is

   a. resorcinol.

   b. benzoyl peroxide.

   c. chlorhexidene (Hibiclens).

   d. pHisoHex.

3. Mrs. P. has an abscessed tooth and has been using a half-strength solution of hydrogen peroxide to rinse her mouth. What instructions will you give her?

   a. Open lesions can occur with chronic use of hydrogen peroxide.

   b. Hydrogen peroxide is very drying to the mucous membranes. Only use it once a day.

   c. Hydrogen peroxide is irritating and can cause bleeding of the gums.

   d. Prolonged use of hydrogen peroxide as a mouthwash can cause you to develop "hairy tongue."

4. The physician orders acyclovir (Zovirax) for an initial outbreak of genital herpes. Which of these instructions should you give the client?

   a. Apply topically to the lesions six times a day for 7 days.

   b. Wash your perineal area before each application and use the medication in the morning and at bedtime.

   c. You should leave the medication on for an hour, then remove it with soap and water.

   d. Apply the medication *no* more than once a day. Overuse will cause severe inflammation.

5. Miss P., age 15, is using benzoyl peroxide for acne. She asks you why she developed acne. Your best response would be

   a. "It is because of your Italian lineage."

   b. "Foods high in fat and caffeine can aggravate acne."

   c. "Emotional stress has been linked to the development of acne."

   d. "Increased secretion of hormones at puberty is a common cause of acne."

6. The physician prescribes isotretinoin (Accutane) for severe cystic acne. An adverse effect of excessive administration of this medication is

   a. atrophy of the skin.

   b. superinfection.

   c. hypervitaminosis A.

   d. loss of pigmentation in the area of the application.

7. This agent is the drug of choice for treating warts.

   a. Silver nitrate.

   b. Acetic acid.

   c. Gentian violet.

   d. Zinc oxide.

8. Which of these medications would be most helpful to relieve itching associated with chicken pox?

   a. Coal Tar (Balnetar).

   b. Colloidal oatmeal (Aveeno).

   c. Trioxsalen (Trisoralen).

   d. Sutilains (Travase).

9. Mr. J. is being treated with topical corticosteroids. You should assess him for

   a. hyperglycemia.

   b. facial lesions.

   c. hair loss.

   d. facial swelling.

10. Which of the following statements by Mr. R. leads you to believe that he has understood the teaching you have done regarding Retin-A?

    a. "I will apply the medication three times daily for 6 weeks."

    b. "My skin may become red and irritated from the medication."

    c. "I will soak my face in cold water before each application."

    d. "This medication will increase my tolerance to sunlight."

CRITICAL THINKING CASE STUDY

M., a 19-year-old college student, comes to the clinic to be treated for acne. She was previously treated at age 16 with tetracycline with limited success. The physician starts her on tretinoin (Retin-A).

1. Identify what instructions you will give M.

M. returns 1 month later. Her facial acne is worse. She states that she has started taking birth control pills.

2. Identify the teaching that you will do with M.

Three months after she has received the medication, M. returns. Her face is excoriated and draining clear serous fluid.

3. Identify what you will do.

67

Drug Use During Pregnancy and Lactation

CHECKLIST

Contraindicated Drugs

Place an × next to the drugs that should be avoided during pregnancy.

1. _____ Captopril (Capoten).

2. _____ Thiazide diuretics.

3. _____ Penicillins.

4. _____ Aminoglycosides.

5. _____ Tetracyclines.

6. _____ Corticosteroids.

7. _____ Laxatives.

8. _____ Oral antidiabetic agents.

9. _____ Quinidine (Quinaglute).

10. _____ Antimanic agents.

11. _____ Alcohol.

12. _____ Nicotine.

MATCHING EXERCISE

Drugs and Indications

Identify the medications that fit the following descriptions.

1. _____ Stimulate uterine contraction; used to initiate the birth process.

2. _____ Causes relaxation of uterine smooth muscle.

3. _____ Used to stimulate labor when uterine contractions are weak and ineffective.

4. _____ The drug of choice for treating pain during labor.

5. _____ Used after delivery of the baby if bleeding is severe.

6. _____ Administered to prevent asthma attacks.

7. _____ Used to treat anemia of pregnancy.

8. _____ The drug of choice for constipation during pregnancy.

9. _____ Used to treat hypertension associated with pregnancy.

10. _____ Intravenous medication that prevents seizures in preeclamptic mothers.

A. Terbutaline (Brethine).

B. Meperidine (Demerol).

C. Ergonovine maleate (Ergotrate).

D. Albuterol (Proventil).

E. Oxytocin (Pitocin).

F. Prostaglandins.

G. Morphine.

H. Magnesium sulfate.

I. Apresoline.

J. Metamucil.

K. Ferrous sulfate.

FILL IN THE BLANKS

Complete the following sentences and phrases.

Vascular System

1. *Normal pregnancy:* Cardiac output _____ 30–40% above the nonpregnant level at approximately the 24th week of gestation.

2. *Normal pregnancy:* A _____% _____ in circulating blood volume occurs because an _____ in plasma renin levels stimulates the secretion of aldosterone, causing retention of Na^+ and H_2O.

3. *Normal pregnancy:* Physiologic _____ develops because of hemodilution of the blood volume.

4. *Normal pregnancy:* Decreased peripheral resistance. There is dilation of the arterial system, causing pooling of blood. Therefore, BP does not go up even though there is a substantial _____ in blood volume.

5. *Pregnancy-induced hypertension:* Hypovolemia occurs despite fluid retention because the fluid shifts into the interstitial space, causing _____.

6. *Pregnancy-induced hypertension:* Decreased platelet count and intravascular coagulation can result in _____.

7. *Pregnancy-induced hypertension:* Increased peripheral resistance and vasoconstriction, leading to increased _____.

Renal System

1. *Normal pregnancy:* _____ glomerular filtration rate (GFR): up to 50% increase to clear creatinine, urea, and uric acid more quickly.

2. *Pregnancy-induced hypertension:* _____ glomerular filtration rate: therefore, increased levels of uric acid (which are associated with poor fetal outcome).

3. *Pregnancy-induced hypertension:* _____ protein loss, _____ Na^+ and H_2O, and _____ urinary output.

Gastrointestinal System

1. *Normal pregnancy:* _____ peristalsis.

2. *Normal pregnancy:* _____ abdominal pressure.

CROSSWORD PUZZLE

Across

3. Parenteral analgesic used during labor.
5. Helpful for treating heartburn.
6. Administered to the mother for its therapeutic effect on fetal tachycardia.
7. Antiemetic used for severe nausea and vomiting.
8. Possible side effects of this drug include hypotension and water intoxication.

Down

1. Analgesic for minor aches and pains during pregnancy.
2. Used to treat chronic hypertension.
4. Used to treat diabetes during pregnancy.

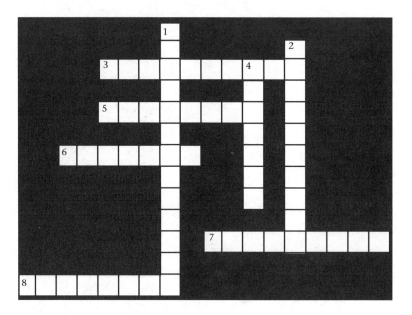

REVIEW QUESTIONS

1. Mrs. J. is 6 months pregnant and her physician tries to stop her labor with ritodrine (Yutopar). Which of the following maternal assessments will you do on an ongoing basis?

   a. Lung sounds.
   b. Hourly urinary outputs.
   c. Deep tendon reflexes.
   d. Level of consciousness.

2. An adverse effect associated with the administration of large doses of oxytocin (Pitocin) is

   a. respiratory distress.
   b. chest pain.
   c. convulsions.
   d. hyperglycemia.

3. The physician orders 4 gm of magnesium sulfate in 250 ml of D5W to infuse over 4 hours. If you administer 1 gm per hour, how fast will you run the IV?

   a. 63 ml/hour.
   b. 78 ml/hour.
   c. 82 ml/hour.
   d. 100 ml/hour.

4. Mrs. G. has epilepsy and is taking phenytoin (Dilantin) and phenobarbital. She is presently 4 weeks pregnant and she is concerned about the effect of the medications on the baby. Identify your response.

   a. "You have nothing to worry about. You are in the hands of a very competent doctor."

   b. "The doctor will probably discontinue your medications until you deliver."

   c. "You should abort this fetus because the medications have already done irreversible damage."

   d. "Maternal ingestion of these drugs may cause neonatal bleeding during the first 24 hours after birth. The baby will receive vitamin K immediately after birth."

5. Mrs. G. is 2 months pregnant and is complaining of nausea. Which of the following instructions will you give her?

   a. "Ask your doctor for an antiemetic."

   b. "Try dry crackers upon awakening. Usually the nausea goes away; if it doesn't, let your physician know."

   c. "Antacids will help; take them as often as you like."

   d. "Constipation makes nausea worse. Mineral oil is very effective in preventing constipation."

6. Mrs. G. develops pneumonia during her pregnancy. Which of the following antibiotics is the safest for use during pregnancy?

   a. Penicillin.

   b. Aminoglycoside.

   c. Tetracycline.

   d. Sulfonamide.

7. Mrs. G. has been taking amitriptyline (Elavil) for depression and asks you about becoming pregnant. The best response to Mrs. G.'s inquiry is

   a. "There have been reports of congenital malformations and neonatal withdrawal when pregnant women take this drug."

   b. "You can use this drug if you discontinue it 1 month before delivery."

   c. "I recommend that you do not become pregnant."

   d. "There are studies that show growth retardation after birth in infants of mothers who take this drug during pregnancy."

8. Which of the following antihypertensive drugs is commonly used during pregnancy and is considered safe?

   a. Hydralazine (Apresoline).

   b. Guanabenz (Wytensin).

   c. Captopril (Capoten).

   d. Clonidine (Catapres).

9. Mrs. J. is receiving a magnesium sulfate drip. Which of the following assessments would indicate toxicity?

   a. Absence of deep tendon reflexes.

   b. A 40-point drop in blood pressure.

   c. Respiratory rate of 36.

   d. Urinary output of greater than 400 ml in 1 hour.

10. You prepare an IV of 1000 ml D5W with 10 units of oxytocin. The drip is started at 2 milliunits per minute. The physician's order is to increase the oxytocin 1 milliunit every 20 minutes. If you are using micro drip tubing (60 drops = 1 ml), by how many drops will you increase the rate of the infusion every 20 minutes?

    a. 2 drops.

    b. 6 drops.

    c. 10 drops.

    d. 12 drops.

CRITICAL THINKING CASE STUDY

Mrs. J. is brought to the hospital. She has been leaking amniotic fluid for 2 days, and her physician has decided to induce her. He orders a prostaglandin vaginal suppository, to be followed by an oxytocin (Pitocin) drip. Mrs. J. is extremely apprehensive and asks why she must receive these medications.

1. Describe how you will respond to Mrs. J.

Two hours after the initiation of the oxytocin drip, Mrs. J. complains of severe pain.

2. Identify what your nursing actions will be.

The physician orders meperidine (Demerol) IV push. During administration of the analgesic, Mrs. J. states that everything is going black and she appears to faint.

3. Identify and prioritize your nursing actions.

Appendix

Drug Calculations

1. Order: Give 1300 mg of calcium carbonate.

   Available: 648 mg/tablet.

   Administer: _____ tablets.

2. Order: Give 250 mg of Diocto-Liquid.

   Available: 50 mg/5 ml.

   Administer: _____ ml.

3. Order: Give 2 tsp of Phanatuss cough syrup.

   Administer: _____ ml.

4. Order: Give 0.3 ml of SSKI.

   Available: 1 gm/ml.

   Administer: _____ mg.

5. Order: Give 400 mg of Tagamet.

   Available: 300 mg/5 ml

   Administer: _____ ml.

6. Order: Give 650 mg of acetaminophen.

   Available: 160 mg/5 ml.

   Administer: _____ ml.

7. Order: 1000 ml D5W to run for 12 hours.

   Available: Tubing that delivers 10 drops = 1 ml.

   Delivery rate: _____ ml/hour.

   Delivery rate: _____ drops/minute.

8. Order: 3 liters of IV solution to run for 24 hours.

   Available: Tubing that delivers 15 drops = 1 ml.

   Delivery rate: _____ ml/hour.

   Delivery rate: _____ drops/minute.

9. Order: 250 ml of D5W at 30 ml/hr.

   Available: Tubing that delivers 60 drops = 1 ml.

   Delivery rate: _____ drops/min.

10. Order: 1000 ml of D5W with 10 mEq KCl over 10 hours.

    Available: KCl 60 mEq/30 ml vial; tubing that delivers 20 drops = 1 ml.

    Inject into IV bag: _____ ml.

    Delivery rate: _____

    drops/minute.

11. A liter of IV fluid is started at 9 A.M. and is to run for 8 hours. The IV is discontinued at 1 P.M.

    How much fluid is left? _____
    ml.

12. Order: IV (piggyback) of gentamycin in 50 ml D5W over 20 minutes.

    Available: Macrodrop set (10 drops = 1 ml).

    Delivery rate: _____

    drops/minute.

13. Order: Heparin sodium 3000 U SC.

    Available: Heparin sodium 10,000 U/ml.

    Administer: _____ ml.

14. Order: Demerol 75 mg, Atropine 0.25 mg IM, Vistaril 12.5 mg.

    Available: Demerol 50 mg/ml, Atropine 0.4 mg/ml, Vistaril 25 mg/ml.

    Administer: _____ ml Demerol.

    Administer: _____ ml Atropine.

    Administer: _____ ml Vistaril.

    Can these medications be administered in the

    same syringe? _____.

15. Order: Phenytoin 75 mg IV.

    Available: Phenytoin (Dilantin) 250 mg/5 ml.

    Administer: _____ ml.

16. Order: Aminophylline 300 mg PO.

    Available: 500 mg/20 ml.

    Administer: _____ ml.

17. Order: Heparin 20,000 units in 1000 ml D5W at 50 ml/hour.

    Delivery rate: _____ units/hour.

18. Order: Nitroprusside 100 mg in 250 ml D5W at 50 ml/hour.

    Delivery rate: _____ mg/hour.

19. Order: Nitroprusside 50 mg in 250 ml D5W at 100 mcg/minute.

    Delivery rate: _____ ml/hour.

20. Order: Dopamine 400 mg in 250 ml D5W at 320 mcg/minute.

    Delivery rate: _____ ml/hour.

21. Order: Norepinephrine 2 mg in 250 ml D5W at 25 ml/hour.

    Delivery rate: _____ mcg/hour.

22. Order: Dobutamine 1000 mg in 500 ml D5W at 20 ml/hour.

    Delivery rate: _____ mg/hour.

23. Order: Dobutamine 250 mg in 250 ml of D5W at 20 ml/hour.

    Delivery rate: _____

    mg/minute.

24. Order: Lidocaine 1 gm in 250 ml D5W at 2 mg/minute.

    Available: Micro drip tubing (60 drops = 1 ml).

    Delivery rate: _____

    drops/minute.

25. Order: Dopamine 400 mg in 500 ml D5W at 60 ml/hour.

    Delivery rate: _____ mg/hour.

26. Order: Isoproterenol 5 mg in 500 ml D5W at 50 ml/hour.

    Delivery rate: _____ mg/hour.

27. Order: Aminophylline 250 mg in 500 ml D5W at 25 ml/hour.

    Delivery rate: _____ mg/hour.

28. Order: Regular insulin 100 units in 250 ml D5W at 30 ml/hour.

    Delivery rate: _____ units/hour.

29. Order: Lidocaine 1 gm in 1000 ml D5W at 60 ml/hour.

    Delivery rate: _____
    mg/minute.

30. Order: Streptokinase 750,000 units in 50 ml over 30 minutes.

    Delivery rate: _____
    units/minute.

ANSWERS

CHAPTER 1

Matching Exercise

Terms and Concepts

1. D.	2. E.	3. A.	4. G.	5. B.
6. K.	7. I.	8. F.	9. H.	10. C.
11. J.	12. O.	13. L.	14. M.	15. N.

Fill in the Blanks

Cell Physiology, Part I

1. Cell membrane.
2. Cytoplasm.
3. Lysosomes.
4. Nucleus.
5. Chromatin.
6. Endoplasmic reticulum.
7. Ribosomes.
8. Golgi apparatus.
9. Mitochondria.

Cell Physiology, Part II

1. Drug movement and therefore drug action are affected by a drug's ability to cross cell membranes.

Review Questions

1. a.	2. c.	3. c.	4. c.	5. d.
6. a.	7. a.	8. d.	9. b.	10. c.

CHAPTER 2

Fill in the Blanks

1. cross cell membranes.
2. Lipid, water.
3. Dosage.
4. slows.
5. lungs, mucous membranes
6. adequacy of circulation.
7. protein binding.
8. unbound.
9. blood–brain barrier.
10. Metabolism.
11. enzymes, liver.
12. enzyme induction.
13. kidneys, bowel, lungs, skin.
14. enzymes, proteins.
15. bind, pharmacologic.
16. number of receptor sites.
17. chemical structure.
18. administration, absorption, distribution.
19. neonates, infants, liver, kidney.
20. tachyphylaxis.

Definitions

1. Movement of a drug from an area of higher concentration to an area of lower concentration.

2. Drug molecules move from an area of lower concentration to an area of higher concentration.
3. The elimination of a drug from the body.
4. The time required for the serum concentration of a drug to be decreased by 50%.
5. Drugs that produce effects similar to those produced by naturally occurring hormones, neurotransmitters, and other substances.
6. Drugs that inhibit cell function by occupying receptor sites.
7. Results when two drugs are taken together, producing a greater effect than when either drug is taken alone.
8. An unexpected reaction to a drug taken for the first time.

Matching Exercise

Terms and Concepts

1. B.	2. C.	3. D.	4. A.

Review Questions

1. c.	2. d.	3. b.	4. b.	5. c.
6. c.	7. b.	8. d.	9. b.	10. a.

CHAPTER 3

Matching Exercises

Terms and Concepts

1. B.	2. F.	3. A.	4. C.	5. D.
6. E.	7. G.	8. H.	9. I.	10. J.
11. L.	12. O.	13. M.	14. N.	15. P.
16. R.	17. K.	18. S.	19. U.	20. V.

Abbreviations

1. I.	2. F.	3. G.	4. C.	5. J.
6. E.	7. B.	8. D.	9. H.	10. A.

Equivalents

1. E.	2. C.	3. H.	4. K.	5. A.
6. D.	7. B.	8. F.	9. G.	10. L.

Diagram

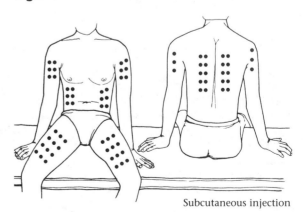

Subcutaneous injection

Practice Questions

Medication Orders

1. b.   2. a.   3. c.

Dosage Calculations

Practice Set I

1. 2 tablets.
2. 0.25 ml.
3. 60 ml.
4. 3 tablets.
5. 0.5 cc.
6. 0.4 cc.
7. 1.25 ml.
8. 8 cc.
9. 4 ml.
10. 0.5 cc.

Practice Set II

1. 60 ml.
2. 3 tablets.
3. 360 ml.
4. 60 kg.
5. 1250 ml.
6. 2.5 ml.
7. 1.2 gm.
8. 0.4 ml.
9. 0.25 ml.
10. 2 tsp.

Review Questions

Dosage Calculations

1. a.   2. a.   3. d.   4. b.   5. c.
6. a.   7. a.   8. b.   9. b.   10. b.

CHAPTER 4

True or False

1. T.   2. F.   3. T.   4. T.   5. T.
6. F.   7. T.   8. T.   9. F.   10. T.
11. T.   12. F.   13. T.   14. T.   15. T.

Review Questions

1. c.   2. d.   3. b.   4. c.   5. d.
6. a.   7. b.   8. b.   9. d.   10. b.

CHAPTER 5

Fill in the Blanks

1. brain, spinal cord.
2. synapse, neurons.
3. acetylcholine, catecholamines (norepinephrine), histamine, serotonin, endorphins, enkephalins.

4. conscious processes.
5. heat, cold, pain, muscle position sense.
6. body temperature, arterial blood pressure, anterior pituitary hormones, food and water intake.
7. cardiac, respiratory, vasomotor.
8. wakefulness, alertness.
9. behavior, emotions.
10. muscular activity, balance, posture.
11. skeletal muscle.
12. medulla.
13. hypoxia.
14. confusion, dizziness, convulsions, loss of consciousness, brain damage.
15. Thiamine.
16. myelin sheaths, Wernicke–Korsakoff.
17. drowsiness, decreased muscle tone, decreased ability to move, decreased perception of sensation.
18. unconsciousness, respiratory failure, death.
19. wakefulness, alertness, decreased fatigue.
20. hyperactivity, excessive talking, nervousness, insomnia.
21. seizures, dysrhythmia, death.

Neurotransmission, Part I

1. Synapse.
2. Release site.
3. Postsynaptic nerve terminal.
4. Receptor sites.
5. Postsynaptic nerve cell membrane.
6. Presynaptic nerve cell membrane.
7. Neurotransmitters.
8. Presynaptic nerve terminal.

Neurotransmission, Part II

1. synapse, receptors.
2. receptor sites.

Review Questions

1. c.   2. b.   3. d.   4. d.   5. a.
6. d.   7. a.   8. c.   9. a.   10. d.

CHAPTER 6

Fill in the Blanks

1. a. Drowsiness and unconsciousness.
   b. Decreased mental and physical activity.
   c. Respiratory depression.
   d. Nausea and vomiting.
   e. Pupil constriction.
2. slowing motility, constipation.
3. PO, IM, IV.
4. 20 mg, 30 mg.
5. Skin patch, 3 days.
6. ASA, Tylenol.
7. short acting, less smooth muscle spasm, 50–100 mg, 2–4 hours.
8. Stadol, Nubain, Talwin.
9. Narcan.
10. assess the patient's pain.
11. ambulation, heat or cold, relaxation.
12. pain threshold, placebo response, behavioral response.

13. IV, it is faster acting.
14. PCA pump.
15. 48 hours.
16. Atropine.
17. crying, thrashing, muscle rigidity.
18. respiratory.
19. smoke, ambulate.
20. Morphine, vasodilation, decreases, decreases.
21. respiratory depression, hypotension, sedation, vomiting.
22. alcohol.

Word Scramble

1. Fentanyl.
2. Codeine.
3. Demerol.
4. Dilaudid.
5. Morphine.
6. Stadol.
7. Darvon.
8. Nubain.
9. Narcan.
10. Talwin.

Word Find

See below.

Review Questions

1. d.	2. a.	3. b.	4. a.	5. d.
6. a.	7. b.	8. d.	9. d.	10. c.

CHAPTER 7

Matching Exercise

Terms and Concepts

1. D.	2. E.	3. A.	4. I.	5. H.
6. B.	7. G.	8. C.	9. F.	10. K.

True or False

1. T.	2. F.	3. F.	4. T.	5. T.
6. T.	7. T.	8. F.		

Review Questions

1. d.	2. a.	3. d.	4. c.	5. b.
6. a.	7. a.	8. b.	9. b.	10. c.

CHAPTER 8

Fill in the Blanks

1. Severe or prolonged.
2. Phobias, panic, obsessive-compulsive, posttraumatic stress syndrome, atypical anxiety disorders, general anxiety.
3. (Rapid eye movement), mentally and emotionally restorative.
4. Pain, anxiety, illness, changes in lifestyle, drugs.

Chapter 6 Word Find

```
N O T H S B H Y P O F T I L C L C E F G H H J N K
K A D R E N E R G I C E N B E T A Z O L O L A N E
C M R I A S S A N L L X Q K E Z S V C D N C A T V
X Y Z T I P L D N E D R O N O N I R L A R N V R R
H L P O D I L A U D I D I C A Y Y O D A V V P P J
F N V A N L I C B R E E K X F H T G N A E S O S B
R I L U A A C A I D D U K L O E E U U E T O R R P
X T O S H R F R N O H A Z Y P X D K B B L K A O T
L R N A Y J R E C L N O S T Y H P E A N B E R E C
V A S G O N I Q P F E N T A N Y L K I S N L O K C
X T K X T G A A N G N P A P E C O R N I U O U S A
K J K X C Z A B T N T A D P V C D T E G F G X H O
V A S D I P I O C P R A Q Z O I N J K A J K L D N
O N A E S O R P T I O N L W N C I N U C N C I V O
P T O M I I A N G I N Y B W I X K U N L S I N E T
A Z A E Y B I D L E S X F N I N S V D F H I A N I
R S C R F X Z Y N G R H V T G N J N A A E Z H T L
G E M O R P H I N E V K O N M H C H L O R Z I D E
Y N O L G D B P Q E R R O T V S P Q Y L O V B P C
L W I E F I C D L S N E V H O W G Y O Z A J O W D
F D O M R G G L I I S T P R O T E R E N E R Z N X
N C O E U M A D I N S F T P T M I G J F U W T C Y
E F D D Q C N Q N T A T D Y M N S J Z E B G O G C
```

5. Benzodiazepines, barbiturates.
6. Liver cells, enzyme induction.
7. Physical, psychological.
8. Fat, plasma proteins.
9. Long, 5–7.
10. (BuSpar), sedation, physical, psychological, muscle relaxant, anticonvulsant.
11. (Vistaril), antiemetic, antihistamine.
12. Chloral hydrate, safe, inexpensive, tolerance.
13. Diphenhydramine (Benadryl).
14. Antianxiety, hypnotic, anticonvulsant, agitation, delirium tremens.
15. Severe respiratory disorders, severe liver disease, hypersensitivity reactions, drug abuse.
16. Increased anxiety, insomnia, irritability, headaches, tremor, palpitations, agitation, confusion, abnormal perception of movement, depersonalization, psychosis, seizures.
17. Flumazenil (Romazicon).
18. Oxazepam (Serax), lorazepam (Ativan).

Nursing Diagnosis

Nursing Diagnosis

1. Sleep pattern disturbance, insomnia.
2. Ineffective individual coping.
3. Knowledge deficit related to the appropriate use of antianxiety medication.

Assessment Data

1. Observe for physiological manifestations of anxiety: increased BP, pulse, respirations, and muscle tension.
2. a. Assess level of anxiety.
   b. Assess effects of anxiety on perception, ability to learn, and problem solving.
3. Assess for a therapeutic response to the medication.

Nursing Interventions

1. a. Reduce environmental stimuli.
   b. Use measures to increase comfort.
   c. Administer antianxiety medication.
2. a. Remain calm.
   b. Assist client to identify stressors.
   c. Provide outlets for excess energy.
   d. Identify previous coping mechanisms.
3. a. Instruct client to avoid alcohol while using the medication.
   b. Instruct client that antianxiety medications are for short-term use.
   c. Assess client knowledge regarding the medications.

Definition

1. A response to a stressful situation resulting in fear, apprehension, nervousness, or worry.

Review Questions

1. d.	2. b.	3. a.	4. c.	5. a.
6. b.	7. a.	8. c.	9. c.	10. c.

CHAPTER 9

Fill in the Blanks

1. Psychosis.
2. Hallucinations.
3. Delusions.
4. schizophrenia.
5. Schizophrenia.
6. phenothiazines.
7. CNS depression, autonomic nervous system depression, antiemetic effect, lowering of body temperature, hypersensitivity reactions.
8. dopamine.
9. anxiety, agitation, hyperactivity, insomnia, aggressive/combative, hallucinations.
10. nausea, vomiting.
11. (Phenergan), sedative, antiemetic, antihistaminic.
12. (Taractan), (Navane), antipsychotic.
13. (Haldol), high, hypotension, sedation, high, extrapyramidal effects.
14. mental retardation with hyperkinesia, Tourette syndrome, Huntington disease.
15. acute dystonia, parkinsonism, akathisia, tardive dyskinesia.
16. (Loxitane), (Clozaril), agranulocytosis, sedation, orthostatic hypotension.
17. Tourette syndrome, tardive dyskinesia, major motor seizures, sudden death.
18. alleviate symptoms, increase the client's ability to cope, promote optimal functioning.
19. respond to another, equivalent.
20. injections, fluphenazine (Prolixin).
21. once, 1–2 hours.
22. 60 ml, fruit juice, water.
23. hypotension, tachycardia, dizziness, faintness, fatigue.
24. dry mouth, caries, blurred vision, constipation, paralytic ileus, urinary retention.
25. menstrual irregularities, possibly impotence, decreased libido, weight gain.

Caution or Contraindication

1. ci.	2. ci.	3. ci.	4. ca.	5. ca.
6. ci.	7. ca.	8. ca.	9. ci.	10. ci.
11. ca.	12. ci.	13. ci.		

Word Scramble

1. Tindal.
2. Mellaril.
3. Compazine.
4. Prolixin.
5. Thorazine.
6. Trilafon.
7. Sparine.
8. Stelazine.
9. Moban.
10. Orap.
11. Clozaril.
12. Haldol.
13. Taractan.
14. Navane.
15. Loxitane.

Word Find

See below.

Review Questions

1. d.	2. d.	3. c.	4. b.	5. b.
6. a.	7. b.	8. c.	9. d.	10. d.

CHAPTER 10

Fill in the Blanks

1. a. Fatigue.
   b. Indecisiveness.
   c. Difficulty concentrating.
   d. Loss of interest in appearance.
   e. Loss of interest in work.
   f. Loss of interest in sex.
   g. Feelings of guilt.
   h. Change in appetite.
   i. Sleep disorder.
   j. Somatic symptoms.
   k. Obsession with death.
2. environmental stress, adverse life events, concurrent disease states.
3. sedation, orthostatic hypotension.
4. (Elavil), TCAs.
5. foods, drugs, hypertensive crisis.
6. tyramine.

7. a. Cheese.
   b. Alcohol.
   c. Bananas.
   d. Caffeine.
   e. Chocolate.
   f. Raisins.
   g. Sour cream.
   h. Yogurt.
8. (Prozac), nausea, nervousness, insomnia, skin rash.
9. (Eskalith), bipolar affective disorder.
10. Adequate kidney function.
11. sodium.
12. several months.
13. a lifetime.
14. 4.
15. 0.8–1.2.
16. 2–3.
17. dry mouth, constipation, blurred vision, tachycardia, orthostatic hypotension, drowsiness, dizziness, excessive.
18. severe nvd (nausea, vomiting, and diarrhea), ataxia, incoordination, dizziness, slurred speech, blurred vision, tinnitus, muscle twitching, tremors, increased muscle tone.

Sentence Correction

1. Urinary retention; *circle* insomnia.
2. Meperidine (Demerol); *circle* Furosemide (Lasix). **Or:** Adrenergic agents, alcohol, guanethidine, levodopa, and reserpine.
3. Sodium; *circle* potassium.
4. Daily; *circle* b.i.d.

Chapter 9 Word Find

5. Severe headaches; *circle* Blurred vision.
6. Renal; *circle* hepatic.
7. Norepinephrine and serotonin; *circle* dopamine and acetylcholine.
8. Arrhythmias; *circle* failure.
9. Hemodialysis; *circle* Gastric lavage.
10. Nicotine; *circle* Caffeine.
11. 4; *circle* 8.
12. Mania; *circle* depression.
13. Physostigmine (Antilirium); *circle* Diazepam (Valium).
14. 2; *circle* 6.
15. 12, 6; *circle* 18, 12.

Review Questions

1. d.   2. d.   3. a.   4. d.   5. d.
6. d.   7. b.   8. d.   9. b.   10. c.

CHAPTER 11

Fill in the Blanks

1. brief episode of abnormal electrical activity.
2. type of seizure characterized by spasmodic contractions of involuntary muscles.
3. chronic recurrent pattern of seizures.
4. EEG.
5. developmental defects, metabolic disease, birth injury.
6. cocaine, lidocaine, theophylline.
7. 5–20 µg.
8. (Valium), acute convulsive seizures.
9. Carbamazepine, psychomotor, tonic-clonic, mixed, trigeminal neuralgia.
10. brain surgery, head injury, drug overdose, electrical imbalance.
11. life long.
12. weeks or months.
13. normal saline, precipitate.
14. Ethosuximide (Zarontin).
15. folic acid.

True or False

1. T.   2. F.   3. F.   4. T.   5. F.
6. F.   7. T.

Crossword Puzzle

Across

2. Klonopin.
4. Tranxene.
5. Valium.
9. Phenobarbital.

Down

1. Convulsion.
3. Tegretol.
6. Dilantin.
7. Depakene.
8. Epilepsy.
10. Ativan.

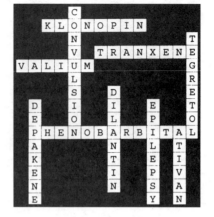

Review Questions

1. a.   2. a.   3. b.   4. b.   5. c.
6. a.   7. a.   8. d.   9. c.   10. c.

CHAPTER 12

Fill in the Blanks

1. chronic, progressive, degenerative, tremor, bradykinesia, joint and muscle rigidity.
2. dopamine, acetylcholine.
3. levodopa, (Lodosyn), (Symmetrel), (Parlodel).
4. (Symmetrel), dopamine release.
5. postsynaptic dopamine receptors.
6. glaucoma, gastrointestinal obstruction, prostate hypertrophy, neck obstruction, myasthenia gravis.
7. most effective.
8. recurrence.
9. Sinemet, brain.
10. (Symmetrel), 1–5.
11. prolong the effectiveness, required dose.
12. bradykinesia, rigidity.

True or False

1. F.   2. T.   3. T.   4. F.   5. F.
6. F.

Review Questions

1. d.   2. d.   3. b.   4. c.   5. a.
6. c.   7. d.   8. a.   9. b.   10. a.

CHAPTER 13

Fill in the Blanks

1. decrease muscle spasms, spasticity.
2. Dantrolene (Dantrium).
3. hyperthermia.
4. mental alertness, physical coordination.
5. baclofen (Lioresal).

6. Diazepam, (Valium), methocarbamol, (Robaxin), orphenadrine citrate, (Norflex).
7. a. Massage, moist heat, and exercise.
   b. Bed rest for acute muscle spasm.
   c. Relaxation techniques.
   d. Correct posture and lifting.
8. Children under 12.
9. 2 mg/minute, respiratory depression and apnea.
10. (Robaxin), bradycardia, hypotension, dizziness.

True or False

1. T.   2. F.   3. F.   4. T.   5. T.

Crossword Puzzle

Across

2. Dizziness.
3. Baclofen.
4. Chlorphenesin.
6. Spasticity.
8. Dantrolene.
9. Pregnancy.
10. Methocarbamol.

Down

1. Massage.
5. Orphenadrine.
7. Diazepam.

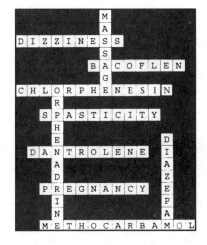

Review Questions

1. a.   2. d.   3. d.   4. a.   5. b.
6. d.   7. a.   8. a.   9. d.   10. d.

CHAPTER 14

Matching Exercise

Terms and Concepts

1. B.   2. A.   3. E.   4. C.   5. I.
6. K.   7. H.   8. G.   9. D.   10. F.
11. L.   12. M.   13. N.   14. P.   15. R.

Word Scramble

1. Ethrane.
2. Forane.
3. Alfenta.
4. Innovar.
5. Pavulon.
6. Anectine.
7. Metubine.
8. Sulfenta.
9. Versed.
10. Brevital.

Word Find

See below.

Review Questions

1. b.   2. d.   3. d.   4. a.   5. a.
6. c.   7. c.   8. d.   9. a.   10. a.

CHAPTER 15

Matching Exercise

Terms and Concepts

1. B.   2. C.   3. E.   4. G.   5. A.
6. F.   7. I.   8. D.   9. H.   10. J.
11. K.   12. M.   13. L.   14. O.   15. N.

Nursing Diagnosis

Nursing Diagnosis

1. Alteration in nutrition: malnutrition and vitamin deficiencies.
2. Risk for violence related to altered thought process.
3. Decreased cardiac output associated with fluid volume excess.
4. Risk for injury related to bleeding.

Assessment Data

1. Lab studies to assess for anemia and electrolyte imbalances. Assess client for signs/symptoms of a deficiency.
2. Assess client for impaired motor coordination, poor task performance, and hypo/hyperactivity.
3. Assess heart sounds, lung sounds, and ECG. Assess lab studies and serum albumin levels.
4. Assess platelet count and clotting studies.

Nursing Interventions

1. Administer folic acid, thiamine, and vitamin B_{12}.
2. Administer sedative. Decrease environmental stimuli. Teach nondrug coping techniques.
3. q4h vs, peripheral pulses. Administer diuretics if appropriate. I & O, daily weights.
4. Observe client for bruising.

Chapter 14 Word Find

```
B A E C C T R I S O M E T A L C H E M P N I P A N
A L T B A C I T R E M E N A R C H O R O L A C O L
C M H T R A L C O H V P E R A G A R I R I H O K C
F O R A N E R L L S S N E S S T I T H E O P H Y L
T S A N S E I O E A A A N I N N O V A R E A N I X
O C N E T I P N E L A T I E N T G E O M T R I C U
B A E A L N P A L P I T F T I O N S E C O E S N E
A N E B O N D I H E X L L G H A L A B F I N I A X
C N U C T E C H Y P A V U L O N V E R E F L E X E
K A P T A B R A P P R E M E N E I O N T A O V A N
H A H S O M T R E M O R A N G C N E J T A O C N I
A B O T P E P I R N N Q B B A T T R I P C O C T N
N C R V Q T I H T E A B I E F I A R E S T L Y H H
E N I M O R B O E H T C N X O N T S E N I M A I C
C I A N S A N T N T A I N T M E T U B I N E M N Y
T A Y N A Z I T S L A E M O R D N F S S E T T E R
O M A H V O T R A C O M M R E X N E O E I F I N T
P P T A M L R T O P A M I N E C T N L B G N O I S
A H A A D Q I C N A A F N N F D D T O E V E S O I
N A T I N V E R S E D I F A E L A A M M P A L O C
T I R E E S T L E S S N E S S U A A W I T O O M
R R F R C S E T R E O N P I I A U N U T W R I M C
Y B B L R S H N V R R S I S E N I K R E P Y H C A
X T E L B E J Q U T H Y P O A C E B R S H I S P W
A L B E L L A D O W D Y M N T E S O O T Y P A K T
```

Definitions

1. A chronic, progressive, potentially fatal disease characterized by physical dependence and physiologic changes related to the ingestion of alcohol.
2. Feelings of satisfaction and pleasure from taking a drug.
3. Physiologic adaption to chronic drug use resulting in uncomfortable symptoms when the drug is stopped.

10. analgesia, migraine headaches.
11. neonates.
12. tolerance, psychological dependence, habituation
13. caffeine.
14. weight, height.
15. excessive CNS stimulation, cardiovascular, gastrointestinal.

Review Questions

1. c.   2. a.   3. d.   4. c.   5. b.
6. c.   7. b.   8. d.   9. d.   10. a.

Review Questions

1. b.   2. c.   3. a.   4. b.   5. c.
6. d.   7. a.   8. d.   9. c.   10. b.

CHAPTER 16

Fill in the Blanks

1. narcolepsy, ADHD (attention deficit-hyperactivity disorder).
2. a rare disorder characterized.
3. children, hyperactivity, a short attention span, difficulty completing assigned tasks, restlessness, impulsive behavior.
4. mood elevation, increased mental alertness, heart rate, blood pressure, mydriasis, gastrointestinal motility, tolerance, dependence.
5. respiration, seizures.
6. mental alertness, drowsiness.
7. cardiovascular disease, anxiety, agitated states, glaucoma.
8. (Ritalin), 6–8.
9. (Dopram), 5–10.

CHAPTER 17

Fill in the Blanks

1. Dilates.
2. Increases.
3. Decreases.
4. Constricts.
5. Increases.
6. Constricts.
7. Contracts.
8. Constricts.
9. Dilates.
10. Decreases.
11. Increases.
12. Dilates.
13. Decreases.
14. Relaxes

True or False

1. T.	2. T.	3. F.	4. F.	5. F.
6. F.				

Review Questions

1. c.	2. d.	3. c.	4. a.	5. b.
6. b.	7. a.	8. b.	9. c.	10. c.

CHAPTER 18

Matching Exercise

Terms and Concepts

1. C.	2. D.	3. A.	4. F.	5. E.
6. B.	7. I.	8. G.	9. H.	10. J.

True or False

1. T.	2. F.	3. F.	4. T.	5. T.
6. T.	7. F.	8. F.	9. T.	10. T.

Sentence Correction

1. Isoproterenol (Isuprel); *circle* Ephedrine.
2. Anaphylactic; *circle* allergic.
3. Allergens; *circle* toxins.
4. Acidosis; *circle* Alkalosis.
5. 30; *circle* 5.
6. Epinephrine; *circle* Levarterenol (Levophed).
7. Stokes–Adams; *circle* Marfan.
8. Phenylephrine; *circle* Pseudoephedrine.
9. Tachycardia; *circle* bradycardia.
10. Under; *circle* over.
11. Blood pressure; *circle* breathing.
12. Rebound nasal congestion; *circle* hypertension.
13. Urinary output; *circle* respiratory status.
14. Increase; *circle* decrease.
15. Hypotension and shock; *circle* bronchodilation and vasoconstriction.

Review Questions

1. b.	2. a.	3. a.	4. b.	5. c.
6. c.	7. a.	8 a.	9. a.	10. c.

CHAPTER 19

Matching Exercise

Terms and Concepts

1. E.	2. F.	3. A.	4. D.	5. B.
6. C.	7. I.	8. G.	9. H.	10. J.

True and False

1. T.	2. T.	3. T.	4. F.	5. T.
6. T.	7. F.	8. T.	9. T.	10. F.

Sentence Correction

1. Propranolol (Inderal); *circle* Nadolol (Corgard).
2. Selective; *circle* nonselective.
3. Supraventricular tachycardia; *circle* hypertension.
4. Timolol (Timoptic); *circle* pindolol (Visken).
5. Propranolol (Inderal); *circle* levobunolol (Betagan).
6. Labetalol (Trandate); *circle* Metoprolol (Lopressor).
7. Atenolol (Tenormin); *circle* penbutolol (Levatol).
8. Nonselective; *circle* Selective.
9. Propranolol (Inderal); *circle* levobunolol (Betagan).
10. Alpha-adrenergic blocking agents; *circle* Beta-adrenergic blocking agents.
11. Decreasing; *circle* increasing.
12. Beta$_1$; *circle* beta$_2$.
13. Bradycardia; *circle* tachycardia.
14. Lipid; *circle* water.
15. Decreased; *circle* increased.

Review Questions

1. a.	2. c.	3. d.	4. c.	5. d.
6. a.	7. d.	8. c.	9. a.	10. d.

CHAPTER 20

Fill in the Blanks

1. a. decreased.
   b. increased.
   c. relaxation of.
   d. increased.
   e. increased.
   f. increased.
   g. constriction of.

Matching Exercise

Terms and Concepts

1. D.	2. A.	3. B.	4. C.	5. E.

True or False

1. T.	2. F.	3. F.	4. T.	5. T.

Review Questions

1. a.	2. c.	3. a.	4. b.	5. c.
6. a.	7. d.	8. d.	9. d.	10. d.

CHAPTER 21

Fill in the Blanks

1. acetylcholine, parasympathetic.
2. a. CNS stimulation followed by CNS depression.
   b. slowed heart rate.
   c. bronchodilation and decreased respiratory tract secretion.
   d. antispasmodic effect in GI tract.

  e. mydriasis and cycloplegia.
  f. decreased secretion of sweat glands.
  g. relaxation of ureters and bladder.
  h. relaxation of smooth muscle of gall bladder and bile ducts.
3. peptic ulcer disease, gastritis, pylorospasm, diverticulitis, ileitis, ulcerative colitis.
4. examination, surgery, mydriatic, cycloplegic.
5. increase.
6. inhalation.
7. increase bladder capacity.
8. respiratory secretions, vagal stimulation.
9. prostatic hypertrophy, glaucoma, tachyarrhythmias, myocardial infarction, CHF.
10. prototype, IM, IV, SC, topically, inhalation.
11. spasm, increased secretion, increased motility.
12. motion sickness, skin patch, 72.
13. Trihexyphenidyl, parkinsonism, extrapyramidal reactions.
14. Benztropine, acute dystonic reactions.
15. dysuria, urgency, frequency, pain.
16. (Ditropan), bladder capacity, frequency.
17. a. gastrointestinal disorders
    b. genitourinary disorders
    c. ophthalmic disorders
    d. respiratory disorders
    e. bradycardia
    f. Parkinson Disease
    g. prior to bronchoscopy
18. physostigmine salicylate, (Antilirium).
19. facial flushing, skin rash
20. blurred vision, confusion, heat stroke, constipation, urinary retention, hallucinations, psychotic-like symptoms.

True or False

1. F.	2. T.	3. F.	4. F.	5. F.

Matching Exercise

1. C.	2. D.	3. A.	4. B.	5. E.
6. F.				

Review Questions

1. c.	2. d.	3. c.	4. c.	5. d.
6. d.	7. a.	8. c.	9. a.	10. b.

CHAPTER 22

Matching Exercise

Terms and Concepts

1. D.	2. E.	3. F.	4. I.	5. J.
6. A.	7. B.	8. G.	9. C.	10. H.
11. L.	12. K.			

True or False

1. T.	2. F.	3. T.	4. F.	5. T.

Review Questions

1. d.	2. a.	3. b.	4. b.	5. a.
6. d.	7. b.	8. b.	9. a.	10. a.

CHAPTER 23

Matching Exercise

Terms and Concepts

1. F.	2. A.	3. D.	4. I.	5. H.
6. L.	7. G.	8. B.	9. C.	10. E.
11. J.	12. K.			

Fill in the Blanks

1. Anterior pituitary.
2. Prolactin.
3. Growth hormone.
4. TSH.
5. ACTH.
6. Posterior pituitary.
7. ADH.
8. Oxytocin.
9. LH.
10. FSH.

Review Questions

1. d.	2. c.	3. d.	4. b.	5. b.
6. b.	7. d.	8. c.	9. d.	10. c.

CHAPTER 24

True or False

1. F.	2. F.	3. F.	4. F.	5. T.
6. T.	7. T.	8. T.	9. F.	10. T.
11. T.	12. T.	13. T.	14. T.	15. F.
16. T.	17. T.	18. F.		

Checklist

Undesirable Effects of Drug Administration

1.	2. ✓	3. ✓	4. ✓	5. ✓
6. ✓	7.	8. ✓	9. ✓	10. ✓
11. ✓	12. ✓	13. ✓	14. ✓	15. ✓
16. ✓	17. ✓	18.	19.	20. ✓
21. ✓	22. ✓	23.	24. ✓	

Word Scramble

1. Vanceril.
2. Celestone.
3. Florinef.
4. Aerobid.
5. Aristospan.
6. Cortef.
7. Medrol.
8. Sterane.

9. Cortone.
10. Decadron.
11. Haldrone.
12. Aristocort.
13. Hydeltrasol.
14. Deltasone.

Word Find

See below.

Review Questions

1. D.	2. B.	3. D.	4. C.	5. D.
6. C.	7. D.	8. A.	9. D.	10. A.

CHAPTER 25

Fill in the Blanks

1. iodine.
2. metabolism.
3. growth, development.
4. poor growth and development, lethargy and inactivity, feeding problems, slow pulse, subnormal temperature, constipation.
5. myxedema, variable depending on amount of thyroid hormone production.
6. nervousness, emotional instability, restlessness, anxiety, insomnia, hyperactive reflexes.
7. tachycardia, fever, dehydration, heart failure.
8. antithyroid drugs, radioactive iodine, surgery, a combination of methods.

9. Levothyroxine (Synthroid), one time, 0.1–0.2 mg.
10. hyperthyroidism.
11. propranolol, (Inderal).
12. 0.08–0.20 mg/100 ml, 5–12 μg/100 ml.
13. 12.
14. height, weight.
15. 100.

Nursing Diagnosis

Nursing Diagnosis

1. Altered nutrition: less than body requirement.
2. Altered bowel elimination: diarrhea.
3. Altered comfort related to hypermetabolic state.
4. Knowledge deficit: related to drug therapy.
5. Altered cardiac output.

Assessment Data

1. Assess weight.
2. Assess for electrolyte imbalance.
3. Assess nutrition.
4. Assess client's knowledge of medication.
5. Monitor vital signs. Observe for symptoms of CHF.

Nursing Interventions

1. Provide extra calories.
2. Instruct to increase fluids. Instruct to avoid foods that cause diarrhea.
3. Instruct to take cool baths and wear lightweight clothing. Instruct to rest.
4. Instruct client regarding antithyroid drugs.
5. Administer propranolol (Inderal) if appropriate.

Chapter 24 Word Find

```
A P P L H E X N O T H S B H Y P O F T I L C L C E
B F G H D J K A D R E N E R G I C E N B E C T A Z
C O L A E N E C M R A I S S A N L L X Q K O V Z S
D E A N L V C D N C H T N H X Y Z T I P L R D N E
E G G H T D R O E O N I R Y L A R N V R H T L P O
F O N T A D I L N C A Y Y D O D A V P P J O F N V
A N L E S C B R E I K X F E H T G N A E B N O S B
R I F L O R I N E F L U A L A C A A I D A E U K L
O E E U N R E T O R P M X T T O S H R F R N O H A
Y P X C E L E S T O N E D R K B B L K A O T L R N
A J R E C L N O N O T D H A R I S T O C O R T S B
H Y P O F T I L C L C R E S F G H H J N K K A D R
E N E R G I C E L N B O E O T D A Z O L O L A N E
C M R A I S S I A N E L L L X E K V Z S X C W C A
H L P O D I R L A U D I D N A C A Y Y O D A U P J
R I L U A E C A A I D A V H A L D R O N E H A P
D K B E C L A O T L R N A Y J D R E C L N O S T Y
M P E N A M B E R E C V A S G R O N I Q P P F E N
T A A E R O B I D N Y L K I G O N L O K C T K X T
G V A A N G A R I S T O S P A N T A P E S C O R N
I U O U S A L E T M O D T I I B T U D H T R P P L
A S O N B S O R P H Y D R O C O C O R T E F I O N
C W A C I N U C N K I X O P T O R I T A R N G I N
Y B P I X K U N L S I N E T A X A A Y B A I D L E
S F N D N S V D F H C I A N I G E M O R N P H A N
K O N M H L O R Z I D E G D E P E R R T E S P L O
```

Definitions

1. Enlargement of the thyroid gland resulting from iodine deficiency.
2. Occurs as the result of a poorly functioning thyroid gland and results in poor growth and development in children.
3. A condition resulting from hypofunctioning of the thyroid gland.
4. A complication of thyrotoxicosis, symptoms of which include severe tachycardia, fever, dehydration, heart failure, and coma.

Review Questions

1. b.	2. d.	3. a.	4. d.	5. c.
6. a.	7. c.	8. b.	9. b.	10. b.

CHAPTER 26

Fill in the Blanks

1. parathyroid hormone, calcitonin.
2. up, down.
3. a. increases bone breakdown or resorption.
   b. increases absorption of calcium from food.
   c. increases reabsorption of calcium in renal tubules.
4. lowers, bone, serum, rapid, short, long term.
5. foods, exposure to sunlight, serum calcium levels, increasing, mobilizing calcium from bone.
6. (Rocaltrol), daily.
7. calcium, phosphorus.
8. 8.8 mg–10.3 mg/100 ml.
9. a. cell membrane permeability and impulses.
   b. nerve cell excitability and transmission of function.
   c. muscle cell excitation and coupling.
   d. blood coagulation and platelet adhesion.
   e. hormone secretion.
   f. enzyme activity
10. milk, vegetables (broccoli, spinach, kale, mustard greens), seafood (clams, oysters).
11. vitamin D deficiency, high fat diet, presence of oxalic acid from beet greens and chard, alkalinity of intestinal secretions, diarrhea.
12. a. is an essential component of DNA, RNA, and other nucleic acids.
    b. combines with fatty acids to form phospholipids, which are required in the structure of all cell membranes.
    c. forms a phosphate buffer system.
    d. is necessary for cell use of glucose.
    e. is necessary for proper function of B vitamins.
13. neuromuscular irritability, tetany.
14. increases.
15. Chvostek's, Trousseau's.
16. vitamin D.
17. excessive vitamin D, thiazide diuretics, estrogen, lithium.
18. depressant.
19. irreversible damage, impairment of function.
20. lowers.
21. (Lasix), increases.
22. Vitamin D, decreasing.
23. blocking resorption from bone.
24. reabsorption of calcium in renal tubules.
25. 3000–4000.

True or False

1. T.	2. F.	3. T.	4. F.	5. T.

Review Questions

1 a.	2. a.	3. d.	4. a.	5. b.
6. c.	7. d.	8. c.	9. d.	10. d.

CHAPTER 27

Fill in the Blanks

1. a. increases.
   b. decreases.
   c. decreases.
   d. increases.
   e. increases.
   f. decreases.
   g. decreases.

Matching Exercise

Terms and Concepts

1. C.	2. D.	3. F.	4. H.	5. E.
6. I.	7. J.	8. K.	9. M.	10. N.

Crossword Puzzle

Across

5. Glyburide.
7. Isophane.
8. Glipizide.
10. Salicylates.
12. Hypoglycemia.

Down

1. Human.
2. Ketoacidosis.
3. Tolazmide.
4. Acetohexamide.
6. Lipodystrophy.
9. Lipid.
11. Beef.

See puzzle below

True or False

1. T.	2. T.	3. F.	4. T.	5. F.
6. F.	7. T.	8. F.	9. T.	10. T.
11. T.	12. F.	13. T.		

Review Questions

1. a.	2. d.	3. b.	4. b.	5. d.
6. d.	7. c.	8. c.	9. b.	10. b.

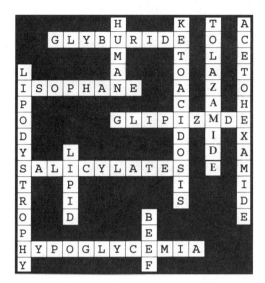

CHAPTER 28

True or False

1. T.	2. F.	3. T.	4. T.	5. T.
6. F.	7. T.	8. F.	9. T.	10. F.
11. T.	12. T.	13. T.	14. F.	15. T.

Fill in the Blanks

1. a. atrophic vaginitis
   b. vasomotor instability
   c. osteoporosis
   d. myocardial infarction

Name that Drug

1. Estradiol transdermal system (Estraderm).
2. Dienestrol (DV).
3. DES (Stilbestrol).
4. Conjugated estrogen (Premarin).
5. Estradiol valerate (Delestrogen).
6. Estradiol cypionate (Depo-Estradiol).
7. Hydroxyprogesterone caproate (Delalutin).
8. Medroxyprogesterone (Depo-Provera).
9. Premarin.
10. Estrogen (Premarin).
11. Oral contraceptives.
12. Estropipate (Ogen).
13. Hydroxyprogesterone caproate (Delalutin).
14. Micronor Nor-Q.D. (Ovrette).
15. Neomycin.

Review Questions

| 1. d. | 2. b. | 3. a. | 4. a. | 5. d. |
| 6. c. | 7. a. | 8. b. | 9. a. | 10. d. |

CHAPTER 29

Circle the Correct Answer

1. increase.
2. increases, decreases.
3. increased.
4. decreases.
5. increase.
6. increase.
7. decrease.
8. increase.
9. decreased.
10. increase.
11. increase.
12. increases.
13. decrease.
14. increase.
15. increase.
16. increase.
17. increase.
18. increase.
19. increase.
20. increase.

Crossword Puzzle

Across

2. Insulin.
3. Electrolyte.
5. Epiphyseal.
6. Halotestin.
7. Testoject.
8. Gonadotropic.
9. Oxandrolone.

Down

1. Danazol.
3. Exogenous.
4. Testosterone.

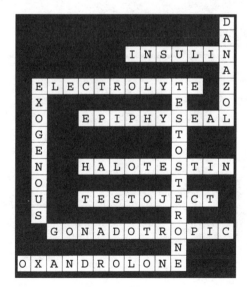

Review Questions

1. b.	2. a.	3. c.	4. d.	5. a.
6. d.	7. d.	8. b.	9. a.	10. b.

CHAPTER 30

Fill in the Blanks

1. P.	2. F.	3. C.	4. P.	5. W.
6. C.	7. W.	8. W, C.	9. F.	10. C, P, F.

True or False

1. F.	2. T.	3. F.	4. T.	5. F.
6. T.	7. F.	8. F.	9. T.	10. F.

Matching Exercise

1. C.	2. B.	3. F.	4. G.	5. E.
6. A.	7. D.	8. J.	9. I.	10. H.

Fill in the Blanks

1. D_5W, 170.
2. 20%, 50%, gluxose hypertonic.
3. 550.
4. water.
5. hypertonic, increase.
6. protein, calories.
7. essential fatty acids, centrally, peripherally.
8. tube placement.
9. 500 ml.
10. 1000.

Review Questions

1. d.	2. a.	3. c.	4. c.	5. c.
6. c.	7. c.	8. d.	9. a.	10. a.

CHAPTER 31

Matching Exercise

Terms and Concepts

1. D.	2. F.	3. H.	4. J.	5. L.
6. A.	7. B.	8. E.	9. I.	10. C.
11. G.	12. M.	13. K.		

Name That Deficiency/Excess

1. Vitamin A deficiency.
2. Vitamin K deficiency.
3. Biotin deficiency.
4. Pyridoxine (vitamin B_6) deficiency.
5. Vitamin C excess, vitamin A deficiency.
6. Severe thiamine deficiency.
7. Vitamin B_{12} deficiency.
8. Severe vitamin C deficiency.
9. Folic acid deficiency, thiamine deficiency.
10. Vitamin A excess.
11. Vitamin C deficiency.
12. Riboflavin deficiency.
13. Niacin deficiency.
14. Vitamin C excess.
15. Vitamin B_{12} deficiency.
16. Vitamin B_{12} deficiency.
17. Vitamin K deficiency.
18. Vitamin A excess.
19. Folic acid deficiency, thiamine deficiency.
20. Vitamin C deficiency.

Review Questions

1. a.	2. b.	3. d.	4. b.	5. d.
6. d.	7. d.	8. a.	9. c.	10. d.

CHAPTER 32

Matching Exercise

Terms and Concepts

1. G.	2. F.	3. D.	4. H.	5. M.
6. I.	7. A.	8. K.	9. B.	10. P.
11. C.	12. E.	13. J.	14. L.	15. O.

Name That Imbalance

1. Hyperkalemia.
2. Zinc deficiency.
3. Hypernatremia.
4. Hypercupremia.
5. Hyperkalemia.
6. Chromium deficiency.
7. Hypokalemia.
8. Hypocupremia.
9. Hyponatremia, hypomagnesemia, hypochloremia.
10. Hemochromatosis.
11. Hypernatremia.
12. Iron deficiency.
13. Hyponatremia.
14. Hypermagnesemia.
15. Hypokalemia.
16. Hyperchloremia.
17. Hypochloremia, hypocalcemia.
18. Hyperkalemia.
19. Hypomagnesemia.
20. Hypermagnesemia.

Review Questions

1. b.	2. b.	3. d.	4. c.	5. b.
6. b.	7. a.	8. c.	9. c.	10. d.

CHAPTER 33

Fill in the Blanks

1. a. breaks in skin.
   b. impaired blood supply.
   c. neutropenia.
   d. malnutrition.
   e. poor hygiene.
   f. suppression of normal flora.
   g. suppression of immune system.
   h. diabetes mellitus.
   i. advanced age.
2. nosocomial.
3. antibacterials, antivirals, antifungals.
4. bactericidal.
5. bacteriostatic.
6. 7–10.
7. reduced, creatinine.
8. aminoglycosides.
9. 1–2 hours, 8.
10. hypersensitivity, superinfection, phlebitis, GI symptoms.
11. a. stomatitis.
    b. diarrhea.
    c. monilial vaginitis.
    d. new localized signs and symptoms, redness, edema.
    e. recurrence of fever and malaise

Review Questions

| 1. b. | 2. a. | 3. c. | 4. c. | 5. d. |
| 6. d. | 7. c. | 8. d. | 9. b. | 10. c. |

CHAPTER 34

Fill in the Blanks

1. streptococcal pharyngitis, pneumococcal pneumonia, gonorrhea, syphilis.
2. respiratory, gastrointestinal, urinary.
3. cloxacillin, dicloxacillin, methicillin, nafcillin, oxacillin.
4. ampicillin.
5. urinary tract, biliary tract, respiratory, ear.
6. ampicillin, sulbactam.
7. carbenicillin, ticarcillin, mezlocillin, piperacillin.
8. gram-positive, gram-negative.
9. first, second, third, fourth.
10. a. respiratory tract.
    b. skin.
    c. soft tissue.
    d. joints.
    e. urinary tract.
    f. bloodstream.
11. meropenem, (Merrem).

Crossword Puzzle

Across

1. Penicillin.
8. Renal.
9. Cerebrospinal.
10. Cefazolin.
11. Augmentin.

Down

2. Ceftriaxone.
3. Prosthetic.
4. Mezlocillin.
5. Tetracyclines.
6. Cefoperazone.
7. Cephalexin.

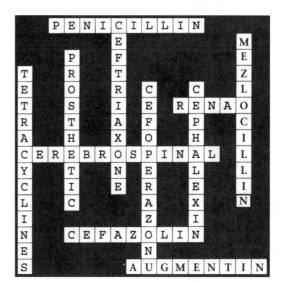

Review Questions

| 1. c. | 2. b. | 3. d. | 4. d. | 5. b. |
| 6. c. | 7. c. | 8. d. | 9. d. | 10. a. |

CHAPTER 35

Fill in the Blanks

1. gram-negative.
2. urinary tract.
3. serious, life-threatening.
4. resistant to other drugs.
5. intestinal bacteria, ammonia.
6. oral, topical, eye, ear, skin.
7. a. check renal function studies.
   b. assess for hearing impairment.
   c. nephrotoxic.
   d. weigh client.
8. serum drug levels, renal function studies, at least 2000–3000 ml.
9. aerobic gram-negative.
10. a. children under 18.
    b. pregnant or lactating females.
    c. those who have had a hypersensitive reaction.
11. 30–60, trough, 10–12, 2.
12. diuretics.

Review Questions

1. b.	2. d.	3. a.	4. b.	5. a.
6. a.	7. b.	8. c.	9. d.	10. d.

CHAPTER 36

Fill in the Blanks

1. gram-positive, gram-negative, rickettsiae, mycoplasmas, protozoa, spirochetes.
2. urine, feces.
3. a. cholera.
   b. granuloma inguinale.
   c. chancroid.
   d. Rocky Mountain spotted fever.
   e. psittacosis.
   f. typhus.
   g. trachoma.
4. Demeclocycline, chronic.
5. mottling of tooth enamel, interfere with bone growth.
6. liver, renal, blood dyscrasia.
7. crystalluria.
8. 1 hour before meals.
9. metallic ions.
10. sunlight, sunburn, skin reactions.
11. bacteriostatic.
12. burn wound infections, ocular, vaginal soft tissue.
13. methoxyflurane, sulfonamides.
14. with, nausea, vomiting, diarrhea.
15. sore mouth, white patches, black furry tongues, diarrhea, skin rash, perineal.
16. milk.
17. 2–3 quarts of fluid daily.

Crossword Puzzle

Across

4. Demeclocycline.
5. Bactrim.
6 Silvadene.

Down

1. Gantrisin.
2. Azulfidine.
3. Sulfamylon.

See Puzzle below.

Review Questions

1. a.	2. d.	3. c.	4. d.	5. d.
6. a.	7. b.	8. d.	9. c.	10. a.

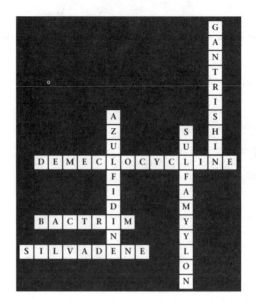

CHAPTER 37

Fill in the Blanks

1. bacteriostatic, high.
2. a. respiratory tract infection.
   b. Legionnaire's disease.
   c. skin infections.
   d. prevention of whooping cough.
   e. as an adjunct to diphtheria antitoxin.
   f. substitute for penicillin.
   g. infections caused by chlamydia.
   h. treatment of intestinal amebiasis.
3. (Zithromax), (Biaxin), respiratory infections.
4. (Chloromycetin), typhoid fever.
5. (Cleocin), streptococcal, staphylococcal, pneumococcal.
6. Vancomycin HCl, (Vancocin).
7. (Flagyl).
8. an empty.
9. nausea, vomiting, diarrhea.
10. nausea, vomiting, abdominal cramps, fever, leukocytosis, abnormal liver function.

True or False

1. T.	2. F.	3. F.	4. T.	5. T.

Review Questions

1. a.	2. a.	3. d.	4. b.	5. c.
6. d.	7. c.	8. c.	9. c.	10. b.

CHAPTER 38

Fill in the Blanks

1. 6.
2. INH, rifampin, pyrazinamide, streptomycin.
3. organisms are resistant to primary drugs.

4. skin test.
5. pyrazinamide, ofloxacin.
6. body weight.
7. 1 hour before, 2 hours after.
8. a. GI problems.
   b. Yellow sclera, dark urine, clay-colored stools.
   c. Changes in hearing or vision.
   d. Numbness or tingling.
   e. Dizziness, drowsiness.
   f. Skin rash or fever.

Matching Exercise

1. E.   2. A.   3. F.   4. B.   5. D.
6. C.

Identify the Treatment

1. A for INH.
2. A for rifampin; C for ethambutol and pyrazinamide.
3. C for pyrazinamide and ofloxacin.
4. C for INH, rifampin, and pyrazinamide.
5. C for INH, rifampin, and pyrazinamide; C* for etham-butol and streptomycin; ✓ for ofloxacin, amikacin, and ciprofloxacin.
6. C for INH, rifampin, and ethambutol.

Review Questions

1. d.   2. a.   3. b.   4. d.   5. c.
6. a.   7. a.   8. d.   9. c.   10. d.

CHAPTER 39

True or False

1. F.   2. F.   3. T.   4. F.   5. T.
6. F.   7. F.   8. F.   9. F.   10. T.
11. F.   12. T.   13. T.   14. T.   15. T.

Matching Exercise

1. E.   2. A.   3. D.   4. B.   5. C.

Review Questions

1. a.   2. b.   3. b.   4. a.   5. d.
6. d.   7. c.   8. b.   9. c.   10. a.

CHAPTER 40

Matching Execise

1. A.   2. G.   3. F.   4. J.   5. I.
6. C.   7. H.   8. E.   9. B.   10. D.
11. O.   12. K.   13. M.   14. N.   15. Q.
16. S.   17. R.   18. T.

Fill in the Blanks

1. inhalation, oral ingestion, implantation.
2. topically.
3. histoplasmosis.
4. candidal.
5. Amphotericin B (Fungizone).

Review Questions

1. b.   2. a.   3. a.   4. b.   5. b.
6. d.   7. d.   8. b.   9. a.   10. b.

CHAPTER 41

True or False

1. T.   2. T.   3. T.   4. F.   5. F.
6. T.   7. T.   8. F.   9. T.   10. F.
11. T.   12. T.   13. T.   14. T.   15. T.
16. T.

Review Questions

1. c.   2. b.   3. c.   4. c.   5. b.
6. a.   7. c.   8. b.   9. c.   10. d.

CHAPTER 42

Matching Exercise

1. D.   2. A.   3. H.   4. J.   5. B.
6. C.   7. E.   8. O.   9. L.   10. F.
11. N.   12. I.   13. G.   14. K.   15. M.

Review Questions

1. c.   2. d.   3. c.   4. a.   5. a.
6. a.   7. a.   8. b.   9. a.   10. d.

CHAPTER 43

Fill in the Blanks

1. antigen, antibody formation, brief, long term.
2. antibodies, a few weeks or months.
3. febrile illness, impaired cellular immunity, leukemia, on steroids, receiving immunosuppressant drugs, pregnancy.
4. 10.
5. cholera, smallpox, yellow fever.
6. temperature.
7. epinephrine.
8. tenderness, redness, Tylenol.
9. paralysis, (Guillain–Barré syndrome).
10. serum sickness, days, weeks.

Exercise on Immunization

Administration of Immunizations

1. SC.   2. IM.   3. PO.   4. IM.   5. SC.

Schedule for Immunization of Infants and Children

See table below.

Review Questions

1. d.   2. c.   3. a.   4. a.   5. d.
6. b.   7. c.   8. a.   9. a.   10. a.

CHAPTER 44

Matching Exercise

1. B.   2. D.   3. F.   4. H.   5. I.
6. G.   7. E.   8. A.   9. J.   10. K.

True or False

1. T.   2. F.   3. F.   4. T.   5. T.

Crossword Puzzle

Across

1. Aldesleukin.
3. Interferon.
4. Neutrophil.
6. Condylomata.
8. Filgrastim.
9. Leukopenia.

Down

2. Sargramostim.
5. BCG.
7. Solid.

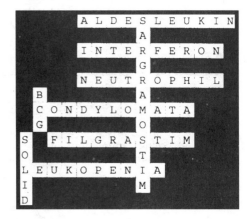

Review Questions

1. a.   2. a.   3. a.   4. c.   5. c.
6. a.   7. d.   8. d.   9. c.   10. c.

CHAPTER 45

True or False

1. T.   2. F.   3. F.   4. F.   5. T.
6. T.   7. T.   8. F.   9. F.   10. F.
11. T.   12. T.   13. F.   14. F.   15. T.

Review Questions

1. a.   2. b.   3. a.   4. a.   5. c.
6. b.   7. c.   8. d.   9. c.   10. b.

CHAPTER 46

Matching Exercises

Terms and Concepts

1. D.   2. E.   3. C.   4. K.   5. F.
6. B.   7. M.   8. I.   9. L.   10. O.

Respiratory System Diagram

1. B.   2. A.   3. D.   4. C.   5. G.
6. E.   7. F.

Review Questions

1. d.   2. b.   3. c.   4. a.   5. d.
6. b.   7. c.   8. a.   9. a.   10. c.

CHAPTER 47

Matching Exercise

1. B.   2. C.   3. D.   4. A.

Fill in the Blanks

1. a. respiratory infections.
   b. odors.
   c. smoke.
   d. cold air.
   e. exercise.
   f. emotional upsets.
   g. tartrazine.
   h. fumes.
   i. drugs.
2. Adrenalin, acute attack of bronchospasm, 5 minutes.
3. Proventil, orally, inhalation.
4. Atrovent, 15, cough, nervousness, nausea, GI upset, headache, dizziness.
5. (Beclovent), (Vanceril), (Azmacort), inhalation.

Schedule for Immunization of Infants and Children

	Birth	1 mo	2 mo	4 mo	6 mo	10–12 mo	15 mo	18 mo	4–6 yr	11–12 yr	Every 10 yr
Polio (OPV)			X	X	X			X	X		
Diphtheria–tetanus–pertussis (DTP)			X	X	X	X		X			
Diptheria–tetanus (DT)										X	X
Measles–mumps–rubella (MMR)							X			X	
Hemophilus influenza Type B (Hib)	X	X	X	X	X		X				
Hepatitis B 1st dose (HBV)	X		X								
Hepatitis B 2nd dose (HBV)		X		X							
Hepatitis B 3rd dose (HBV)					X			X			
HBV, if not previously immunized										*	
Varicella zoster (Var) chicken pox						X		X		†	

(Adapted by Rachel Hofstetter)

Based upon recommendations from the Advisory Committee on Immunization Practices (ACIP), the American Academy of Pediatrics (AAP), and the American Academy of Family Physicians (AAFP).

Arrows indicate that immunization should be done within the marked span of time.

* Series started.

† Unvaccinated children who lack a reliable history of chicken pox should be vaccinated.

6. (Intal), allergic asthma, exercise-induced asthma.
7. confusion, restlessness, anxiety, increased BP, increased pulse.
8. 2000–3000, thin their secretions, nervousness, insomnia.
9. bronchodilator.
10. fungal infection of the mouth and throat.

True or False

1. F.   2. T.   3. T.   4. F.   5. F.

Review Questions

1. d.   2. d.   3. d.   4. d.   5. d.
6. b.   7. d.   8. b.   9. c.   10. a.

CHAPTER 48

Matching Exercise

Terms and Concepts

1. B.   2. C.   3. E.   4. G.   5. A.
6. F.   7. H.   8. J.   9. I.   10. D.
11. L.   12. N.

Review Questions

1. c.   2. a.   3. d.   4. c.   5. b.
6. d.   7. a.   8. d.   9. d.   10. b.

CHAPTER 49

Fill in the Blanks

1. nasal decongestants.
2. profuse discharge from the nose.
3. cough.
4. immobility, cigarette smoking, surgical procedures.
5. rest and sleep.
6. acetylcysteine, (Mucomyst).
7. codeine, hydrocodone, hydromorphone, morphine.
8. rebound nasal congestion.
9. increase.
10. nausea, vomiting, constipation, dizziness, drowsiness, pruritus, drug dependence.
11. MAO inhibitors.
12. blow his or her nose.
13. 20–30 minutes before feeding.
14. 30 minutes.
15. 2000–3000 ml.

Crossword Puzzle

Across

1. Sudafed.
5. Dextromethorpan.
9. Nasal.

Down

2. Acetylcysteine.
3. Acetaminophen.
4. Rhinitis.
5. Dimetapp.
6. Organidin.
7. Robitussin.
8. Antitussives.

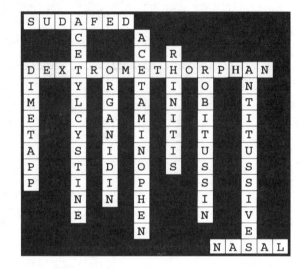

Review Questions

1. c.   2. d.   3. a.   4. a.   5. a.
6. c.   7. a.   8. c.   9. c.   10. a.

CHAPTER 50

Matching Exercise

Terms and Concepts

1. C.   2. A.   3. F.   4. G.   5. J.
6. K.   7. L.   8. N.   9. H.   10. M.

Fill in the Blanks

1. Coronary arteries.
2. Superior vena cava.
3. Right atrium.
4. Tricuspid valve.
5. Inferior vena cava.
6. Right ventricle.
7. Aorta.
8. Pulmonary artery.
9. Left atrium.
10. Mitral valve.
11. Chordae tendon.
12. Papillary muscle.
13. Left ventricle.
14. Septum.

Review Questions

1. a.   2. b.   3. b.   4. b.   5. d.
6. c.   7. c.   8. d.   9. a.   10. c.

CHAPTER 51

Fill in the Blanks

1. increases, increases, vasoconstriction, increases, increases, ventricular hypertrophy.
2. preload.
3. increase, slow.
4. fibrillation, flutter.
5. 0.75–1 mg.
6. 0.1 mg.
7. 0.057 mg.
8. (Inocor), short-term.
9. cardiac arrhythmias.
10. 20–30%.
11. arrhythmias.
12. digitalis effects.
13. digoxin toxicity.
14. a. arrhythmias.
    b. anorexia, nausea, and vomiting.
    c. headache, drowsiness, and confusion.
    d. visual disturbances.
15. a. large doses.
    b. impaired renal function.
    c. age extremes.
    d. hypoxia.

Matching Exercise

Terms and Concepts

1. F.	2. H.	3. K.	4. A.	5. E.
6. G.	7. M.	8. D.	9. J.	10. I.
11. L.				

Review Questions

1. b.	2. c.	3. b.	4. d.	5. b.
6. c.	7. c.	8. a.	9. a.	10. a.

CHAPTER 52

Matching Exercise

Terms and Concepts

1. B.	2. A.	3. F.	4. G.	5. J.
6. M.	7. L.	8. E.	9. D.	10. C.

Crossword Puzzle

Across

9. Digoxin.
10. Disopyramide.

Down

1. Quinidine.
2. Propranolol.
3. Pronestyl.
4. Lidocaine.
5. Quinidine.

6. Atropine.
7. Adenosine.
8. Verapamil.

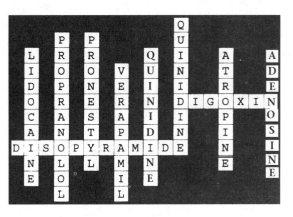

Cardiac Electrophysiology Exercise

Part I: Diagram Completion

1. Left atrium.
2. Left ventricle.
3. Left bundle branch.
4. Purkinje fibers.
5. Right bundle branch.
6. Bundle of His.
7. Right ventricle.
8. AV node.
9. Right atrium.
10. SA node.

Part II: Drug Effects on Cardiac Physiology

1. 7, right ventricle; 2, left ventricle.
2. 10, SA node; 8, AV node.
3. 8, AV node; 6, bundle of His; 5, right bundle branch; 7, right ventricle; 3, left bundle branch; 2, left ventricle.
4. 10, SA node; 8, AV node.

Dysrhythmia Analysis

1. Supraventricular tachycardia, adenosine (Adenocard).
2. Atrial fibrillation, digoxin (Lanoxin).
3. Sinus bradycardia, atropine.
4. Premature ventricular contractions, lidocaine (Xylocaine).

Review Questions

1. b.	2. a.	3. c.	4. b.	5. b.
6. b.	7. c.	8. b.	9. a.	10. b.

CHAPTER 53

Fill in the Blanks

1. venous pressure, venous return to the heart, blood volume, blood pressure (preload), cardiac workload, oxygen demand, flow to the myocardium, peripheral resistance.
2. heart rate, myocardial contractility, blood pressure, myocardial workload, oxygen demand.
3. coronary, peripheral arteries, myocardial contractility.
4. heavy meals, cigarette smoking, strenuous exercise.
5. diet, adequate rest.
6. 5, three, see their physician.
7. hypotension, dizziness, headaches.
8. hypotension, bradycardia, bronchospasm, congestive heart failure.
9. a. ×.
   b. ×.
   c.
   d. ×.
   e.
   f.
   g. ×.
   h. ×.
10. avoid strenuous exercise, assume a supine position.

Matching Exercise

Terms and Concepts

1. E.	2. B.	3. G.	4. A.	5. I.
6. H.	7. K.	8. C.	9. F.	10. L.

Fill in the Blanks

Effects of Nitroglycerin

1. arterioles.
2. venules.
3. peripheral resistance.
4. venous return.
5. afterload.
6. preload.
7. myocardial oxygen demand.
8. angina.

Review Questions

1. d.	2. d.	3. b.	4. b.	5. c.
6. c.	7. a.	8. a.	9. d.	10. c.

CHAPTER 54

True or False

1. F.	2. F.	3. T.	4. T.	5. F.
6. T.	7. F.	8. T.	9. F.	10. T.

Fill in the Blanks

1. decreased, decreased, decreased.
2. peripheral vascular resistance.
3. myocardial contractility, heart rate.
4. 90/60, 50 ml/hour.
5. phentolamine, (Regitine).

Review Questions

1. b.	2. a.	3. a.	4. d.	5. b.
6. b.	7. d.	8. a.	9. a.	10. c.

CHAPTER 55

Matching Exercise

Terms and Concepts

1. E.	2. A.	3. F.	4. B.	5. C.
6. D.	7. G.			

Fill in the Blanks

Cardiovascular Indications for Use

See table below.

Name That Drug

1. Captopril (Capoten).
2. Labetolol (Trandate).
3. Sodium nitroprusside (Nipride).
4. Hydrochlorothiazide (Hydrodiuril).
5. Beta blockers.
6. Beta blockers, calcium channel blockers.
7. Vasodilators.
8. Clonidine (Catapres).
9. Diet and exercise.
10. Antiadrenergic, vasodilators, ACE inhibitors plus loop diuretics.
11. Thiazide diuretics.
12. Reserpine (Serpasil).
13. Clonidine (Catapres), guanabenz (Wytensin).
14. Enalapril (Vasotec), lisinopril (Zestril).
15. Alpha blockers, direct vasodilators.
16. Nonselective beta blockers, propranolol (Inderal).

Review Questions

1. a.	2. d.	3. b.	4. b.	5. a.
6. d.	7. c.	8. d.	9. c.	10. c.

CHAPTER 56

Fill in the Blanks

1. glomerular filtration, tubular reabsorption, tubular secretion.
2. 400 ml, normal amounts, metabolic endproducts.
3. proximal tubule.

4. Antidiuretic hormone, water.
5. Aldosterone, sodium, potassium.
6. uric acid, creatinine, hydrogen ions, ammonia.
7. potassium ions, hydrogen ions, ammonia.
8. a. increased capillary permeability.
   b. increased capillary hydrostatic pressure.
   c. decreased plasma osmotic pressure.
9. tissue fluids, decreasing plasma volume.
10. peripheral vascular resistance, sodium, have a vasodilating effect on arterioles.
11. Thiazide diuretics, 2.
12. sodium, potassium, Hyperkalemia.
13. solute load, (osmotic pressure), water, bloodstream, Mannitol.
14. electrolytes, uric acid, blood glucose, creatinine, BUN.
15. blood pressure, weight, urine output, edematous extremities.
16. digoxin toxicity, diuretic-induced hypokalemia.
17. 3.5–5.0 mEq/L.
18. a. giving supplemental potassium.
   b. giving potassium-sparing diuretic.
   c. increasing potassium intake.
   d. using salt substitutes.
   e. restricting sodium.
19. a. ECG changes.
   b. dysrhythmias.
   c. hypotension.
   d. weak shallow respiration.
   e. anorexia.
   f. nausea, vomiting.
   g. paralytic ileus.
   h. skeletal muscle weakness.
   i. confusion, disorientation.

True or False

1. F.	2. T.	3. T.	4. F.	5. F.
6. F.	7. F.	8. F.	9. T.	10. F.

Fill in the Blanks

The Nephron

1. Efferent arteriole.
2. Afferent arteriole.
3. Bowman's capsule.
4. Glomerulus.
5. Distal tubule.
6. Proximal tubule.
7. Collecting tubule.
8. Descending limb of loop of Henle.
9. Ascending limb of loop of Henle.
10. Loop of Henle.

Review Questions

1. c.	2. c.	3. d.	4. a.	5. b.
6. a.	7. b.	8. c.	9. b.	10. c.

Chapter 55 Fill in the Blanks

	Angina pectoris	Hypertension	Arrhythmias	Heart failure	MI
Amlodipine (Norvasc)	X	X			
Enalapril (Vasotec)		X		X	
Diltiazem (Cardizem)	X	X*			
Felodipine (Plendil)		X			
Nifedipine (Adalat, Procardia)		X*			
Verapamil (Calan, Isoptin)	X	X	X		
Captopril (Capoten)		X		X	
Propranolol (Inderal)	X	X	X		X
Metoprolol (Lopressor)		X			X
Esmolol (Brevibloc)			X		

* Only the sustained release formulations (diltiazem SR and nifedipine SR) are approved for treatment of hypertension.

CHAPTER 57

Fill in the Blanks

Drug Interactions

1. Increase.
2. Increase.
3. Decrease.
4. Decrease.
5. Increase.
6. Decrease.
7. Increase.
8. Increase.
9. Decrease.
10. Decrease or increase.

Drug Indications and Actions

Heparin

1. Acute thromboembolic problems, prophylaxis for clients at risk following administration of thrombolytic agents.
2. Rapid, within minutes.
3. Short.
4. IV, SC.
5. Activated partial thromboplastin time (APTT).
6. Protamine sulfate.

Coumadin

1. Long-term treatment for prevention of clot formation.
2. Delayed 2–5 days.
3. 2–5 days after discontinuation.
4. PO.
5. Prothrombin time (PT) and International Normalized Ratio (INR).
6. Vitamin K.

Streptokinase

1. To dissolve thrombi and limit tissue damage.
2. Immediate.
3. Minutes after discontinuation.
4. IV.
5. Thrombin time (TT), activated partial thromboplastin time (APTT), prothrombin time (PT).
6. Amicar.

Review Questions

1. b.	2. b.	3. b.	4. c.	5. d.
6. c.	7. c.	8. a.	9. a.	10. c.

CHAPTER 58

Matching Exercise

Terms and Concepts

1. C.	2. B.	3. D.	4. A.	5. F.
6. E.				

Fill in the Blanks

Treatment of Hyperlipidemia

See table below.

Review Questions

1. c.	2. b.	3. c.	4. d.	5. a.
6. d.	7. a.	8. a.	9. d.	10. b.

CHAPTER 59

Matching Exercises

Terms and Concepts

1. D.	2. E.	3. F.	4. G.	5. A.
6. I.	7. K.	8. B.	9. C.	10. M.
11. N.	12. O.	13. P.	14. Q.	15. R.

Digestive System Diagram

1. G.	2. C.	3. A.	4. B.	5. E.
6. D.	7. F.			

Review Questions

1. b.	2. a.	3. c.	4. c.	5. c.
6. d.	7. b.	8. b.	9. c.	10. d.

CHAPTER 60

Matching Exercise

Terms and Concepts

1. B.	2. C.	3. D.	4. A.	5. E.
6. F.	7. I.	8. H.	9. G.	10. J.

True or False

1. T.	2. F.	3. F.	4. F.	5. F.
6. F.	7. T.	8. F.	9. T.	10. T.

Fill in the Blanks

1. reflux esophagitis, gastritis, heartburn.
2. gastric acid.
3. amount, acidity.

4. potent, drug interactions.
5. Pepcid, Axid, mental confusion, gynecomastia.
6. Cytotec, GI bleeding.
7. Carafate, ulcer, coating, healing.
8. a. cigarette smoking.
   b. physiological stress.
   c. psychological stress.
   d. genetic influences.
   e. sex.
   f. drug therapy.

Matching Exercise

1. D.   2. F.   3. C.   4. G.   5. E.
6. B.   7. H.   8. A.

Crossword Puzzle

Across

1. Misoprostol.
4. Sodium.
9. Calcium.
10. Hypersecretion.

Down

2. Prostaglandins.
3. Palatability.
5. Cimetidine.
6. Aluminum.
7. Omeprazole.
8. Sucralfate.

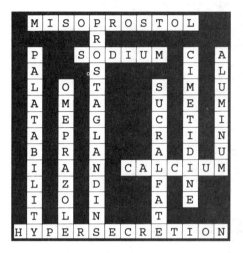

Review Questions

1. b.   2. c.   3. c.   4. c.   5. b.
6. b.   7. a.   8. b.   9. d.   10. a.

Chapter 58 Fill in the Blanks

Treatment	Hyperlipidemia					
	I	IIa	IIb	III	IV	V
Cholestyramine (Questran)		X				
Pravastatin (Pravachol)		X	X			
Gemfibrozil (Lopid)					X	X
Nicotinic acid (Niacin)		X	X	X	X	X
Colestipol		X				
Lovastatin (Mevacor)		X	X			
Diet modification	X	X	X	X	X	X
Exercise	X	X	X	X	X	X

CHAPTER 61

Matching Exercise

Terms and Concepts

1. F.	2. E.	3. A.	4. D.	5. G.
6. B.	7. H.	8. C.	9. I.	10. J.
11. L.	12. N.	13. O.	14. Q.	15. P.

Definitions

1. Laxatives that decrease the surface tension of the fecal mass and allow water to penetrate.
2. The elimination of feces from the colon.

Review Questions

1. a.	2. d.	3. c.	4. a.	5. b.
6. a.	7. c.	8. a.	9. a.	10. c.

CHAPTER 62

True or False

1. F.	2. T.	3. T.	4. T.	5. F.
6. T.	7. T.	8. F.	9. T.	10. F.
11. T.	12. F.	13. F.	14. F.	15. T.

Fill in the Blanks

1. a. intestinal infections.
   b. undigested/coarse/spiced foods.
   c. excessive use of laxatives.
   d. lack of digestive enzymes.
   e. inflammatory bowel disease.
   f. drug therapy.
2. a. replacement fluids (tea, bouillon, jello).
   b. restrict intake.
   c. rest.
   d. avoid foods that irritate the GI mucosa.

Review Questions

1. b.	2. b.	3. a.	4. b.	5. c.
6. d.	7. c.	8. c.	9. b.	10. d.

CHAPTER 63

Matching Exercise

Terms and Concepts

1. J.	2. A.	3. I.	4. B.	5. C.
6. H.	7. D.	8. G.	9. E.	10. F.
11. O.	12. L.	13. N.	14. M.	15. P.

Review Questions

1. a.	2. a.	3. d.	4. b.	5. c.
6. a.	7. c.	8. a.	9. b.	10. b.

CHAPTER 64

Matching Exercise

Terms and Concepts

1. D.	2. J.	3. A.	4. I.	5. B.
6. H.	7. G.	8. F.	9. C.	10. E.
11. L.	12. K.	13. O.	14. M.	15. N.

True or False

1. T.	2. T.	3. F.	4. T.	5. T.
6. T.	7. F.	8. T.	9. T.	10. T.
11. F.	12. T.	13. F.	14. F.	15. T.

Fill in the Blanks

Cell Cycle

1. Mitosis occurs.
2. Resting phase.
3. RNA and enzymes required for the production of DNA are developed.
4. DNA is synthesized for chromosomes.
5. RNA is synthesized and the mitotic spindle is formed.

Review Questions

1. a.	2. a.	3. d.	4. c.	5. b.
6. c.	7. a.	8. a.	9. c.	10. d.

CHAPTER 65

Matching Exercises

1. E.	2. D.	3. C.	4. B.	5. A.
6. J.	7. F.	8. G.	9. I.	10. H.

Fill in the Blanks

1. dilate the pupils.
2. inflammatory conditions.
3. decreases.
4. dye, diagnose.
5. increased intraocular pressure, four, constrict.
6. dilate, glaucoma.
7. weekly, glaucoma.
8. irrigating the eyes with copious amounts of water as soon as possible.
9. trifluridine, (Viroptic).

Name That Drug

1. Osmotic diuretics.
2. Miotics.
3. Anticholinergics.
4. Carbonic anhydrase inhibitors.
5. Adrenergic mydriatics.

Drug Classification

1. Dipivefrin (Propine); *Use:* glaucoma examinations, uveitis, pre- and post-op mydriasis, local hemostasis
2. Timolol maleate (Timoptic); *Use:* glaucoma
3. Pilocarpine (Pilocar); *Use:* glaucoma
4. Physostigmine salicylate (Isopto Eserine); *Use:* glaucoma
5. Atropine sulfate; *Use:* examinations, pre- and post-op uveitis, secondary glaucoma
6. Acetazolamide (Diamox); *Use:* glaucoma, pre-op
7. Glycerin (Osmoglyn); *Use:* pre-op, acute glaucoma
8. Apraclonidine (Iodipine); *Use:* glaucoma, prevention of increased intraocular pressure after ocular surgery
9. Benoxinate hydrochloride (Dorsacaine); *Use:* tonometry, removal of sutures and foreign bodies.
10. Silver nitrate; *Use:* prophylaxis of gonorrhea.
11. Methylcellulose (Methulose); Use: protect cornea during eye exams, keratitis, or wearing contact lenses
12. Latanoprost (Xalatan); *Use:* glaucoma

Review Questions

1. b.	2. a.	3. c.	4. a.	5. c.
6. a.	7. b.	8. b.	9. d.	10. d.

CHAPTER 66

Matching Exercise

Terms and Concepts

1. N.	2. A.	3. M.	4. B.	5. L.
6. C.	7. K.	8. D.	9. J.	10. E.
11. F.	12. I.	13. G.	14. H.	15. O.
16. T.	17. P.	18. S.	19. Q.	20. R.

Review Questions

1. b.	2. a.	3. d.	4. a.	5. d.
6. c.	7. a.	8. b.	9. b.	10. b.

CHAPTER 67

Checklist

Contraindicated Drugs

1.	2. ×.	3.	4. ×.	5. ×.
6.	7.	8. ×.	9.	10. ×.
11. ×.	12. ×.			

Matching Exercise

Drugs and Indications

1. F.	2. A.	3. E.	4. B.	5. C.
6. D.	7. K.	8. J.	9. I.	10. H.

Fill in the Blanks

Vascular System

1. increases.
2. 50, increase, increase.
3. edema.
4. anemia.
5. anemia.
6. increase.
7. BP.

Renal System

1. Increased.
2. Decreased.
3. increased, retention of, decreased.

Gastrointestinal System

1. Decreased.
2. Increased.

Crossword Puzzle

Across

3. Meperidine
5. Antacids
6. Digoxin
7. Dramamine
8. Oxytocin

Down

1. Acetaminophen
2. Methyldopa
4. Insulin

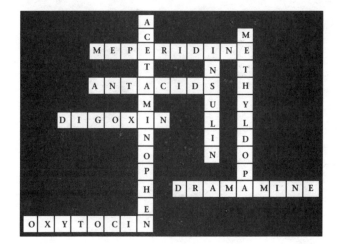

Review Questions

1. a.	2. c.	3. a.	4. d.	5. b.
6. a.	7. a.	8. a.	9. a.	10. b.

APPENDEX

1. 2 tablets.
2. 25 ml.
3. 10 ml.
4. 300 mg.
5. 6.7 ml.
6. 20 ml.
7. 83 ml/hour, 14 drops/minute.
8. 125 ml/hour, 31 drops/minute.
9. 30 drops/minute.
10. 5 ml, 33 drops/minute.
11. 500 ml.
12. 25 drops/minute.
13. 0.3 ml.
14. 1.5 ml Demerol, 0.6 ml Atropine, 0.5 ml Vistaril; yes, these medications can be administered in the same syringe (total volume = 1.5 ml + 0.6 ml + 0.5 ml = 2.6 ml; can use one or two syringes).
15. 1.5 ml.
16. 12 ml.
17. 1000 units/hour.
18. 20 mg/hour.
19. 30 ml/hour.
20. 12 ml/hour.
21. 200 mcg/hour.
22. 40 mg/hour.
23. 0.33 mg/minute.
24. 30 drops/minute.
25. 48 mg/hour.
26. 0.5 mg/hour.
27. 12.5 mg/hour.
28. 12 units/hour.
29. 1 mg/minute.
30. 25,000 units/minute.